THE STORY OF SLEEP

THE STORY OF SLEEP

From A to Zzzz

DANIEL A. BARONE, MD
WITH LAWRENCE A. ARMOUR

ROWMAN & LITTLEFIELD
Lanham • Boulder • New York • London

The information contained in this book is designed to help the reader make informed decisions regarding sleep and wellness. This book is not a medical manual. It is not a replacement for treatment(s) that the reader's personal physician may have suggested. If the reader is experiencing a medical issue, professional medical help is recommended. Mention of particular products, companies, or authorities in this book does not entail endorsement by the publisher or author.

The author gratefully acknowledges the generous support of the innovative sleep company MOLECULE toward the publication of this book.

Published by Rowman & Littlefield
An imprint of The Rowman & Littlefield Publishing Group, Inc.
4501 Forbes Boulevard, Suite 200, Lanham, Maryland 20706
www.rowman.com

86-90 Paul Street, London EC2A 4NE

British Library Cataloguing in Publication Information Available

Library of Congress Cataloging-in-Publication Data
Names: Barone, Daniel A., author. | Armour, Lawrence A., author.
Title: The story of sleep : from A to Zzzz / Daniel A. Barone with Lawrence A. Armour.
Description: Lanham : Rowman & Littlefield, [2023]
Identifiers: LCCN 2022029248 (print) | LCCN 2022029249 (ebook) | ISBN 9781538169735 (cloth) | ISBN 9781538169742 (ebook)
Subjects: LCSH: Sleep—Health aspects—Popular works. | Mind and body—Popular works. | Self-care, Health—Popular works.
Classification: LCC RA786 .B37 2023 (print) | LCC RA786 (ebook) | DDC
    616.8/498—dc23/eng/20220623
LC record available at https://lccn.loc.gov/2022029248
LC ebook record available at https://lccn.loc.gov/2022029249

CONTENTS

ACKNOWLEDGMENTS

First of all, I would like to thank God, who makes all things possible. Thank you to Mom and Dad, for your love and support through the years and for always believing in me. But I'm not sure where you will display this book—the den cabinet is filled!

Thank you to my sister, Laura, my biggest supporter. "Sometimes life can be tough. And I know that sometimes it's hard 'Keeping the Faith'"—but you manage to do so every day. Love ya!

Thank you, Larry Armour, for your enthusiasm, patience, and expertise in making our second book a reality. If you had not convinced me to give it a second go-around, this book would not have happened.

I want to thank Joan Parker for your belief in our little team and for your guidance, as well as your diligence and effort to help us get published a second time.

Thank you to Suzanne Staszak-Silva and all at Rowman & Littlefield Publishing for once again taking a chance on us.

Thank you to Molecule Mattresses and Comfort DTC Inc. for their support not only of myself but also of our writing team. Your mattress and bedding products are second to none, and I am grateful to work with such an integrous and dynamic company.

I would like to express my gratitude to Weill Cornell Medical College, New York-Presbyterian Hospital, the Weill Cornell Center for Sleep Medicine, and all the colleagues and staff members who provide such wonderful service to our patients.

Speaking of which, I want to sincerely thank all of my patients for trusting me with your care and for teaching me the most important lessons about being a doctor.

Last, but definitely not least, I want to sincerely thank my mentors, friends, and loved ones for believing in me along the way—you know who you are! Thank you for your love and support from the bottom of my heart. It means the world to me.

Daniel A. Barone, MD, FAASM, FANA
June, 2022

Be who God meant you to be and you will set the world on fire.

—St. Catherine of Siena

INTRODUCTION

In the introduction to my first book, I wrote that I have always been fascinated by sleep. I also mentioned that my goal in writing *Let's Talk About Sleep* was to share my enthusiasm for the subject and to highlight what I have learned about sleep during my years as a neurologist. If the phone calls, letters, and emails I have received since the publication of the book are any indication, it's clear that many of you not only share my fascination with sleep but are also eager to learn more.

The Story of Sleep: From A to Zzzz is designed to fill that gap by providing additional guidance for those who understand how critical sleep is to their health and who want to do all they can to improve the quality of their sleep. Seeing a physician to ensure that what you are doing is safe is always the best place to begin. And while what is written here will not be the answer for everyone, I hope that it will at least inspire you to examine new approaches that may help you and your loved ones sleep better.

As you will soon see, *The Story of Sleep: From A to Zzzz* is alphabetized. Many of the entries are short and bite-sized. You may find that as you are reading, there are terms or phrases you are not familiar with—and this is okay. I have written the book this way so that you can pick it up at any point, read about a topic that interests you or you want to know more about, and then put it down and start another entry whenever you like. For convenience, you will see a fair number of parenthetical instructions (i.e., "see . . ."), which are there to help this process along. In my own life, I find I get the most out of books that break things up in this manner.

Any discussion of what can be done to improve sleep health must first address what the problems are. That being the case, let's take a moment to look at a few of the main topics we will be addressing in this book.

The most prominent condition patients tell me they would like to improve is insomnia. Depending on the medical literature you read, most people have experienced some form of insomnia at one point or another in their lives, and many experience a chronic form (defined as one that occurs for more than three months). As we get into the subject, you will see that while certain medications and over-the-counter substances *can* be used, the "real" answer lies in improving behaviors and habits long-term.

Another bread-and-butter condition I often see is obstructive sleep apnea (OSA). Best described as a repetitive, temporary stoppage of breathing that occurs throughout the night, OSA can lead to short-term and long-term consequences. We don't usually think of medications as ways to combat OSA, but we often use technology in the form of continuous positive airway pressure (CPAP) machines. It should be noted, however, that in June 2021, Philips, one of the CPAP manufacturers, recalled 3.4 million CPAP machines that were allegedly blowing small particles into the air tubes and then into the lungs of patients, raising concerns of lung irritation and cancer. Since then, the process of replacing these machines has led to a shortage of CPAP machines produced by other manufacturers. I am hopeful that by the time this book comes out, these issues will have been resolved. That said, while most patients do not have a problem with CPAP, many find it uncomfortable or intrusive. Fortunately, there are ways to deal with this, as well as many other options we will discuss throughout the book.

One note on the use of the term "OSA" and "sleep apnea"—there are various forms of sleep apnea, including central sleep apnea (see "Central sleep apnea"). We usually group all forms of breathing problems in sleep under the umbrella term "Sleep-disordered breathing" (see "Sleep-disordered breathing [SDB]"). As you read through this book, you may see "OSA" and "sleep apnea" used interchangeably, and for the most part, they are interchangeable. But just be aware of other types of sleep apnea, with central sleep apnea being the most prominent. When we are discussing central sleep apnea, it will be clearly stated.

Many people have heard about narcolepsy through television and movies, where, unfortunately, it is usually portrayed in a comedic or dramatic way. By definition, narcolepsy is a condition combining unrelenting sleepiness with other symptoms, such as dreams and hallucinations, as people drift into sleep or are about to wake up; it additionally can include sleep paralysis (which is exactly what it sounds like). There may also be present a bizarre phenomenon known as cataplexy. Cataplexy is a loss of muscle tone in the context of a very emotional or funny situation, leading some people to fall or have other embarrassing consequences. The classic way to treat narcolepsy is with medications, but there are other ways to improve sleep and daytime function, which we will get into.

Another condition that is sometimes misunderstood is restless legs syndrome (RLS). This is a condition in which patients complain of an uncomfortable feeling in their legs, which usually comes on around bedtime. By getting up and moving around the bedroom, the symptoms often abate. As you can imagine, this repetitive and annoying phenomenon can inhibit a patient's ability to get to sleep. If that weren't enough, people with RLS can have the "asleep" version, called periodic limb movements of sleep (PLMS). These are, as you can guess, leg (or sometimes arm) movements that occur throughout the sleep period and can disturb the patient's and/or the bed partner's sleep. Fortunately, like the other conditions above, there are ways to treat this—again, mostly with medications, but natural, non-medication regimens also exist that we will be discussing in detail.

Other lesser-known conditions include those related to our circadian rhythm, also known as our internal clock. People can have trouble if their sleep clock is set too early, also known as advanced sleep phase disorder (ASPD), or if it is set too late, it is known as delayed sleep phase disorder (DSPD). In both ASPD and DSPD, there can be disturbances in a person's social and work life. In the case of DSPD, there can be a particularly fruitless and quite disheartening lack of improvement when the condition gets misdiagnosed and is treated as simple insomnia. To that end, as you can guess, there are other things to try either in conjunction with medication or on their own.

Finally, there are habits and behaviors that are not necessarily sleep "diseases," but ones that can impair our ability to sleep well and feel well. I am referring to the usage of electronics, alcohol, other substances, and other forms of stimulation. We will go over all of these and discuss ways to lessen their negative impact on your sleep health.

Although sleep is vital for healthy human functioning, studies show that most American adults get around six hours of sleep per night, which is less than the seven to nine hours per night that most experts say are needed. Studies also suggest that approximately one-third of adults report sleep difficulties, making insufficient sleep one of the most pressing, critical issues of the times.

Insufficient quality or quantity of sleep increases a person's susceptibility to disease and chronic illness. It also harms psychological and cognitive functioning. Regular and sufficient sleep performs a crucial role in maintaining and restoring the human body. At a physiological level, sleep loss can undercut the intake of new knowledge, the repair of skeletal muscles, and the efficient removal of waste from the brain. Insufficient sleep may also affect mood, negatively impact metabolism, and increase systemic inflammation, as well as contribute to a weakened immune system. These aspects of proper sleep have always been vital, of course, but even more so now in the wake of the COVID-19 pandemic.

Before we begin, one item must be mentioned in the interest of full disclosure. Please note that I am a consultant to Molecule, one of the leading producers of mattresses, pillows, and related items. Several of its products are mentioned in the relevant sections of this book.

But enough background—let's get to the specifics.

Accidents. Sleep deprivation is a rampant problem these days, and it's easy to see why. As a society, we sleep one hour less per night than our ancestors. That doesn't sound like much, but it's actually very significant. The average person needs seven to nine hours of sleep per night. If someone who needs eight hours a night is only getting six, this means they have been getting two hours less than they need per night. As a result, after only four nights, they are essentially eight hours "behind." That equates to basically one night a week without sleep, which has a potentially dangerous effect over time: blood pressure is likely to go up, excess inflammation may occur, the risk of catching a cold or other viruses (like COVID-19) goes up, and cardiovascular risk increases.

As for car accidents, we know there's an association between lack of sleep and cognitive performance. Driving requires good reaction time, avoiding risky behavior, and being vigilant. It is well-known that people who are sleep deprived, either from quantity or from things like sleep apnea, are at increased risk for car accidents. Reaction time, judgment, vigilance, and overall decision making may be affected. In fact, studies have shown a disconnect between our subjective feeling of being sleepy compared to our objective impairment; in plain English, we don't realize how sleepy we are at times. An unfortunate example of this is that the Monday after daylight savings time kicks in is the number one day for car accidents in America. As of the writing of this book, the US Senate passed a bill called the Sunshine Protection Act, which would make daylight saving time permanent starting in November of 2023. But that still leaves the problem of sleep deprivation the other 364 days, and car and heavy machinery accidents may be the result.

Acid reflux is also known as gastroesophageal reflux disease (GERD) and/or heartburn. Why does it develop? We breathe in by expanding our chest cavity, which generates negative pressure and causes us to suck in air from the environment. In the case of obstructive sleep apnea (OSA), there is a blockage of the airway—that is, an obstruction typically resulting from the tongue falling backward. When this happens, the chest has to work extra hard to generate negative pressure, which can cause acid to be sucked up from the abdomen. Especially when lying flat, that acid can irritate the esophagus and lead to heartburn. The only clues that a person may have OSA could be coughing at night or frequent awakenings without an explanation. If you have either of these symptoms, talking to your clinician is important. A sleep test might also be useful.

Acupuncture is a form of traditional Chinese medicine in which thin needles are inserted into the body in an attempt to relieve pain as well as improve conditions like insomnia. The theory is based on the ancient Taoist Wuxing, otherwise known as the five elements in the West. The life force energy called *qi*, acupuncturists believe, flows from the organs to the skin, muscles, tendons, bones, and joints through channels called meridians; the acupuncture needles are placed around these meridians. Furthermore, disease is thought to be a disharmony in the energies (such as yin and yang) and in the meridians. The therapeutic approach is to find the pattern of disharmony by looking at aspects of the body such as the color and shape of the tongue, the strength of pulse-point, or the sound of the voice.

As an interesting aside, the logo of the American Academy of Sleep Medicine is the yin/yang symbol. However, treatments such as acupuncture are not listed as recommended in the clinical practice guidelines for the treatment of insomnia. The scientific conclusions of research studies and systematic reviews have been inconsistent as far as determining whether acupuncture is a reliable clinical approach. My belief—and one that I frequently share with patients—is that if a treatment doesn't hurt and it may help, it might be worth a shot.

Acute insomnia is something we have all experienced. The night before a big test or a presentation, we may not be able to get to sleep or stay asleep. Typically, once the stressful event has passed, sleep returns to normal. It is only a serious problem when it becomes chronic (see "Insomnia").

ADHD (attention deficit hyperactivity disorder) is a chronic condition leading to inattention, hyperactivity and impulsivity, difficulty regulating emotions, or problems with cognition. It is an important diagnosis in the sleep world for three reasons: (1) because it can sometimes be the "wrong" diagnosis in a case of narcolepsy or sleep apnea insofar as sleepiness is actually the cause of the inattention, not ADHD itself; (2) it can often co-occur in other sleep disorders such as insomnia; and (3) the medications used to treat ADHD (see "Stimulant medications") can make insomnia worse.

Adenosine is a naturally occurring chemical that relaxes and dilates blood vessels. It has many effects in the human body, and it is used as a treatment in certain heart rhythm disorders. For our purposes here, adenosine builds up over the course of a day and signals the brain that the person is sleepy. Caffeine, a stimulant, stops the adenosine signal from acting. Interestingly, the use of cannabis in rats causes adenosine levels to rise and makes them sleepy.

Advanced sleep phase disorder is a problem stemming from a faulty "internal clock" (see "Circadian rhythm") in which the clock is set too early; patients prefer to get to sleep early and wake early. It is unlike its cousin, delayed sleep phase disorder, in which patients prefer to go to bed late and wake up late. Advanced sleep phase disorder is generally seen in older people, who as an example, would go to bed at eight o'clock in the evening and wake at four o'clock in the morning. We treat this by introducing bright light in the early evening to "trick" the brain to keep melatonin from being released too early, keeping the person awake until a more appropriate time.

Alarm clocks are similar to naps in that they both can be very helpful if used the right way. This may sound a bit strange, but I mean that alarm clocks can help us to stick to a good sleep-and-wake routine, keeping our internal clocks set right. They can also be detrimental to sleep. One thing I find is that many times, people will set the alarm ten to thirty minutes before they want to wake up, so that they can hit the snooze and go back to sleep. This feeling of going back to sleep releases serotonin in the brain, but the brain is not an on-off switch. The process of waking up, then going back to sleep, and then waking up again can leave us feeling "hungover" and suffering from sleep inertia (see "Sleep inertia"). It's better to just set the time you need and get up then. Also, watching an alarm clock throughout the night can worsen insomnia, so I tell my patients to use an alarm clock but to keep it covered or facing away from the bed.

Alcohol and sleep. We've all heard that a nightcap—an alcoholic drink before bed—is good for sleep. But it's more likely that glass of wine or shot of something stronger has a downside we tend to ignore. According to "Why You Should Limit Alcohol Before Bed for Better Sleep," which appeared in the June 17, 2020 issue of the Cleveland Clinic's Health Essentials, a drink of alcohol before bed can cause you to fall asleep more quickly, but the result can be an increase in NREM sleep and a decrease in REM (rapid eye movement) sleep—a combination that can lead to not only intense dreams and nightmares but also an increase in sleep apnea and sleepwalking. Another study by the Sleep Foundation (www.sleepfoundation.org/nutrition/alcohol-and-sleep) concludes that low amounts of alcohol decrease sleep quality by roughly 9 percent, while high amounts tend to decrease the quality of sleep by more than 39 percent. Typically, it takes about two hours for the body to metabolize a drink—whether that be a glass of wine, a shot, or a beer—and I urge people to take that into account. A glass of wine with dinner is fine, but several drinks right before bed can disrupt your sleep that night.

Alpha waves refer to brainwaves seen during a sleep test; we see them most often during the relaxed mental state with eyes closed. Researchers traditionally believed that alpha waves indicate a wakeful period during sleep, which is known as alpha wave intrusion, but this is controversial. The theory is that people who have alpha waves in NREM (non-rapid eye movement) sleep have lower quality sleep, which is associated with conditions like fibromyalgia. This is a phenomenon that is not well understood, and alpha waves themselves may be an essentially normal finding.

Anatomy of sleep. Any discussion of sleep must mention the component parts of our brain, so we can have a better understanding of how the process unfolds. The brain is composed of billions of cells; some are the "brains" of the operation (pun intended) and some do the "supporting" work. Neurons are the cells that process and formulate information, but they are not the only cells that make up the brain's structure. Another type of cell, called astrocytes, carries the burden of housekeeping and yardwork of the brain. These cells help the neurons get the nutrients they need while keeping the bad elements away.

The brain is broken up into four lobes and the cerebellum. The four—frontal, temporal, parietal, and occipital lobes—form the cerebrum, and the cerebellum (it is weird that the names are so similar) is the funny-looking structure located just beneath the occipital lobe. The frontal lobe is the area of the brain located right above the eyes. Its main area of concern is *executive function*, a fancy term for what we do when we plan our day, decide what we are going to do and say, and even what we shouldn't say. This illustrates the important point that the frontal lobes are like a filter for the rest of what the brain wants to do. The left and right frontal lobes control decision making and personality, but there are three other lobes: the temporal lobe, the parietal lobe, and the occipital lobe.

The parietal lobes are located right behind the frontal lobes, basically after the halfway point of the brain. They have many functions related to sensation. As the frontal lobes help control the planning and actual doing of movements, the parietal lobe receives information about what the body is experiencing in terms of simple sensations (such as what your hand touches), to more complex things (such as knowing where your hand is located at any given moment), to even more abstract ideas like "this is my hand and no one else's."

The temporal lobe is located underneath the parietal lobe on each side of the brain. In fact, if you touch your temple, that is the approximate area of your temporal lobe. It has many functions— almost a seemingly random mix of things, to be honest. It has a hand in memory, the sensation of smell, and even the sensation of hearing.

The occipital lobe is responsible for vision and visual processing. It is located in the back of the skull and, interestingly, contains a spatial map of the retinal visual field.

The cerebellum, which lies at the base of the skull, helps us coordinate our movement and speech. In alcoholics, many times the cerebellar structures are damaged, which leads to imbalance and slurred speech in some cases.

Those are the main structures of the brain that are involved in everything we do. There are subsections of these structures that play an important role in sleep, which we will talk about in more detail now.

The internal clock is called the suprachiasmatic nucleus, or SCN for short. Some people have proposed that this collection of cells has its origin in evolution as a sort of transformed eye. It receives signals of light from our retina, and from these signals, it is able to determine if it is a proper time to sleep. Any kind of light, whether from a desk lamp or an overhead ceiling lamp, is sensed by the SCN as a reason to stay awake. It was not wired into our circuitry that there would be artificial light in human history; therefore, the SCN cannot tell whether the light coming to it is from the sun or a lamp, and thus, it keeps us awake because humans are supposed to be awake when there's light.

Once the SCN decides that it is time for bed, it begins to shift certain areas of the brain and brainstem, through a very complex series of circuits, into lower gears. One of the major things it does is to signal the pineal gland to make melatonin. Melatonin, a chemical the brain makes and releases, has a variety of physical consequences. While it has antioxidant effects, its major job is to promote sleep.

The pineal gland is a very interesting structure in the brain and has perplexed and inspired multiple thinkers, religious authorities, and others to decipher its meaning. For example, in ancient Indian tradition, we have a "third eye," which corresponds to the sixth chakra and acts as a window to the spirit world. It is also responsible for the effects of meditation and clairvoyance. Rene Descartes viewed the pineal gland as "the seat of the soul" and the driver of the "human machine" (for more, see "Descartes and the Pineal Gland," https://plato.Stanford.edu).

The 1958 discovery of melatonin, the hormone produced by the pineal gland, demonstrated the effects of the gland on controlling our sleep and wake cycles. Furthermore, it has been discovered that our

DNA contains genes that both literally and figuratively act as clocks which drive the twenty-four-hour rhythms of behavior and physiology; the master clock in this case in the pineal gland.

Anemia is a blood disorder in which the blood has a reduced ability to carry oxygen. If the anemia is chronic it can generate many symptoms that can masquerade as sleep-related issues, including tiredness, weakness, shortness of breath, and headaches. One major cause of anemia is low iron (see "Ferritin"), which can lead to restless legs syndrome (see "Restless legs syndrome [RLS]") and make it much more difficult to treat. Anemia is discovered through simple blood tests. Treatments include curing the underlying cause and/or use of vitamin B12 or iron supplements, depending on the nature of the anemia.

Antidepressants are common medications used to treat major depressive disorder, some anxiety disorders, some chronic pain conditions, and to help manage some addictions. Side effects include dry mouth, weight gain, dizziness, headaches, sexual dysfunction, and emotional blunting. Some antidepressants can worsen sleep or make sleep less deep. Others can improve it and still others can bring on REM behavior disorder and other types of movements in sleep (see "Parasomnias"). While they may affect sleep negatively, antidepressants may absolutely be needed, which is a major reason I recommend many of my patients see a psychiatrist.

Antihistamines are drugs used to treat allergies, nasal congestion, hives, and symptoms of cold or flu. They usually are over the counter and are used for short-term treatment. Since one common side effect of antihistamines is drowsiness (Benadryl is an example), people often take them for sleep. Unfortunately, there are consequences with this in the long term: (1) antihistamines can leave us feeling hungover the next day; (2) we get used to them very quickly, and more and more are required to get the same effect; (3) they can affect memory; and (4) they can make restless legs syndrome much worse. If used every now and then (when you have a cold or flu and need to sleep), antihistamines should not be a problem. In older people, however, they can lead to dizziness/unsteadiness in the middle of the night if used chronically.

Anxiety disorders can come from any number of stressors, including life or work difficulties, which are common and which we have all experienced. Most anxiety disorders, however, are more severe; they are characterized by significant and uncontrollable feelings of anxiety and fear, which can affect a person's social, occupational, and personal functions. They may result in restlessness, irritability, fatigue, problems concentrating, increased heart rate, chest pain, abdominal pain, and, of course, insomnia. When a patient tells me their history and an anxiety disorder is a possible additional problem, I will encourage them to find a psychiatrist or therapist; without treatment, the insomnia will be much more difficult to treat. As an aside, I consider depression disorders and anxiety disorders to be two sides of the same coin.

APAP. An automatic positive airway pressure device (sometimes called AutoPAP and sometimes, AutoCPAP) works by automatically fine-tuning the amount of pressure delivered to the airway in someone who has obstructive sleep apnea. It is essentially a "smart" machine that calibrates the needs of the patient on a moment-to-moment basis. Another plus is that we can get a patient on it without an in-lab titration study as would be required for CPAP.

Apnea. Sleep apnea is a condition that most commonly refers to obstructive sleep apnea (OSA), but there are others such as central sleep apnea—a sleep disorder in which breathing continuously halts and begins during the night. If an individual snores loudly while sleeping or feels fatigued when he or she gets up in the morning, he or she may be one of the 18 million Americans who currently suffer from sleep apnea.

Snoring is an extremely common phenomenon. When someone has a tightened airway—which can come from nasal congestion, a deviated septum, fat tissue around the neck, a genetically tight airway, a large tongue, or a combination of any of the above—the result can be snoring, which is simply a vibration of these tissues. Snoring by its own accord is not considered dangerous but can be associated with OSA.

OSA is very common condition that affects roughly 25 percent of men and 10 percent of women, and these numbers will likely increase given the current obesity epidemic in the United States. It is characterized by repetitive stoppages of breathing caused by the tongue and soft tissues falling backward and literally choking off the airway. By definition, each of these stoppages is ten seconds in length, as determined by a sleep test. The mainstay of treatment for OSA is continuous positive airway pressure, known as CPAP, which provides a continuous stream of pressurized air that acts as an airway splint to prevent not only snoring but OSA as well.

Some people find that CPAP machines are uncomfortable, intrusive, anxiety provoking, or, simply, they just don't want to use them. In these cases, we as a patient-doctor partnership need to do one of a few things. I always recommend giving CPAP a try because it is a treatment that will essentially work in every case. The problem is not "Will this work for my OSA?" Rather, it is "Will I be able to tolerate it?"

To help patients learn to tolerate the CPAP, I suggest that they begin by trying it before bed. If someone watches TV in the evening, I may suggest that they place the CPAP on then and wear it during their TV hours. This is not going to offer any benefit in terms of treatment (sleep apnea only happens *in sleep*), but it will help them get used to the idea, discomfort, and so on. Additionally, in many cases, I find that some "performance anxiety" goes into putting on a CPAP right before bedtime, especially if someone is nervous or anxious about wearing one to be begin with. That fear of "I have to put this on right now and then wear it correctly through the night, and I'm not sure it will work for me . . ." can be lessened by practicing, so to speak, earlier in the day.

Another recommendation for CPAP would be an (approximately) ten-minute session of mindfulness or a guided meditation with the CPAP in place before bed. Again, this would help reduce the potential anxiety or racing thoughts that can sometimes develop when a person puts on a CPAP mask. I, occasionally, will even prescribe sleep medications to help a patient get over the hump when trying a CPAP for the first couple of weeks or months. Also, in the case of "going natural," we can try either melatonin, valerian, or others in conjunction with meditation.

Other treatments for OSA that you will find throughout this book include the mandibular advancement device (MAD, which is otherwise known as an oral or dental device for OSA), nasal expiratory positive airway pressure (nasal EPAP) surgical options, and the Inspire device (and similar products). The bottom line is that OSA is a dangerous condition—not over one night necessarily but over years. Because we know it can lead to heart disease, diabetes, strokes, and so on, it is important to treat it.

Asthma is a common, chronic, inflammatory disease of the airways of the lungs, which leads to episodes of wheezing, coughing, chest tightness, and/or shortness of breath. These symptoms can occur several times per day or a few times per week (or even less); they can get worse at night, but not always. There seem to be genetic and environmental triggers/causes, and untreated sleep apnea may make it worse.

ASV (adaptive servo-ventilation) are special CPAP-type machines that assist to ensure normal breathing. CPAP works by using air pressure to keep the airway wide open. ASV does the same but more. It can detect reductions in breathing and respond with added pressure to maintain a patient's breathing. ASV is used in cases of central sleep apnea (see "Central sleep apnea [CSA]") or complex sleep apnea, which is a type of central sleep apnea that occurs when a person uses CPAP. When someone has congestive heart failure (a major cause of central sleep apnea), we must be cautious in using ASV, as some literature suggests that it can do more harm than good.

Autoimmune diseases are a group of conditions in which the body's immune system essentially attacks itself. Symptoms include a low-grade fever and feeling tired, and in many cases, the cause is unknown. Diseases known to be autoimmune include celiac disease, diabetes mellitus type 1, Graves' disease, inflammatory bowel disease, multiple sclerosis, psoriasis, rheumatoid arthritis, and lupus. Approximately 24 million people in the United States are affected, and women are more commonly affected than men. With regards to sleep, there can be fatigue. Narcolepsy, REM behavior disorder, and insomnia have also been linked to autoimmune conditions.

A form of narcolepsy caused by an autoimmune reaction to the H1N1 flu vaccine appeared during the 2009 winter months, and some literature expresses concern that as the COVID-19 pandemic winds down, it will be followed by an uptick in narcolepsy. In these cases, the concern is that the virus itself would trigger the immune system to recognize certain nerve cells as enemies and thus attack them. Similarly, one of the most feared results of COVID-19 and the vaccine is that of developing Guillain-Barré syndrome, a neurological disorder in which the body's immune system damages nerve cells, causing muscle weakness, or, in the most severe cases, paralysis. Regardless of the type and cause of an autoimmune disease, there are no cures, and treatment is usually given as supportive measures to manage the symptoms.

Bathing. According to a wide variety of studies, a hot bath or shower taken one to two hours before bed helps some people fall asleep a little quicker than normal. Although it sounds counterintuitive, the warm water causes blood to circulate from the core of your body to your hands and feet. Since the core body temperature lowering is a signal for sleep, a warm bath/shower may help get you there.

Bedding/sheets. When it comes to sheets, pillows, mattresses, and other key elements that have an impact on how we sleep, it is important to know all you can about their strengths and potential weaknesses. Anything that can cause discomfort—whether it be itchy fabric or trapped heat—can disturb your sleep. If you find yourself uncomfortable when you wake up, kicking the covers off during the night, or sweating while you sleep, a different set of sheets may be the answer.

While a review of each is beyond the scope of this book, a quick online look at the best in the various categories should tell you what you need to know. In the final analysis, what's most important when it comes to sheets is personal: it could be anything from the color to the cost to the kind of fabric. Are you looking for sheets with a specific feel or, rather, a set of cooling sheets for summer and cozy flannel sheets for cold winter months? Materials are probably the most important component of a sheet set, as seen by manufacturers' use of terms like *100 percent cotton* or *ultra-soft microfiber*.

Bed sheets can cost anywhere from fifteen to twenty to even thousands of dollars, depending on the brand. According to study conducted by *U.S. News & World Report*, the average price is $146. The following description of the types of materials typically found in sheets, compiled by *U.S. News,* provides a summary of what to look for when you decide to invest in new sheets (www.usnews.com/360-reviews/sleep/sheets /best-cooling-sheets).

- *Cotton.* Many sheet sets are made with 100 percent cotton. Long-staple cotton is comprised of durable, longer fibers that intertwine, creating a smoother material that's less likely to pull, because there are fewer exposed ends. The two types of long-staple cotton sheets are Egyptian cotton and Pima cotton.
- *Organic.* When talking about sheets, organic usually refers to plant materials (typically cotton) that are grown without the use of pesticides or other synthetic chemicals.
- *Jersey.* A type of fabric made with a jersey knit. Originally from wool, jersey is now made with cotton, synthetic fibers, and blends and is known for its soft, stretchy feel.
- *Microfiber.* Microfiber is a term given to materials made of extremely thin synthetic fibers, often used in cleaning cloths. It is lightweight and has moisture-wicking properties.
- *Percale.* Percale is a type of fabric weave—threads woven in a pattern of one thread over and one thread under—resulting in a durable fabric with a flat and even finish. These tend to have a crisp feel to them, like a dress shirt. They are also breathable, making them a good choice if you're looking for sheets that let you sleep comfortably cool.
- *Sateen.* Like percale, sateen is a type of weave, rather than a type of raw material, where tiny streaks of threads are all going in the same direction. This leads to fabric with a silky, smooth feel and soft sheen. One thing to note is that sateen tends to trap heat more than percale, so it may not be the best choice for those who already sleep too warm.
- *Flannel.* Not just for plaid shirts, this fabric is heavier and thicker than others you commonly see for sheets. It is most often used in the winter, as it has a cozy feel and traps heat well. It has a thick but relatively loose weave that's brushed to make it slightly fuzzy. Originally made solely from wool, it is now made with cotton, synthetic thread, wool, or a combination.

- *Linen.* Linen is a fabric made from flax. It is absorbent and dries quickly but, more importantly, is very lightweight and breathable. In sheets, its breathability and moisture-wicking properties can be beneficial to those who sleep hot, and it is a good choice for those looking for a natural material.
- *Bamboo.* Viscose, also called rayon, is fabric made from the cellulose of bamboo and other plant materials. Similar to linen, bamboo sheets are breathable and boast moisture-wicking properties.

Bedroom environment. The bedroom should be as dark as you can make it without you hurting yourself. A night light is okay, but nothing more. Black-out shades can shield the light from outside and an early morning sunrise. The bed environment should be as quiet as possible. Ear plugs are great, as is a white noise machine. Sleeping with a fan, an HVAC unit, or an air conditioner can also be fine, provided the sound is a constant low humming ("white noise").

The environment should also be on the cool side—not freezing but cool, in the high sixties or so. The body temperature normally drops in the middle of the night, and that helps to promote deep sleep. If the room or bed is too hot, sheets and mattresses can help cool the body's core temperature as well. Finally, there should be no TV in the room, or access to a computer, video games, and so on. The bed environment should be looked at as a "holy place" where you do your sacred act of sleeping—therefore, anything that would desecrate that holy place should be removed.

These tips should improve your sleep. They will not cure everything, but they are a good place to start.

Bed wetting, also known as enuresis, is the inability to hold urine during the night in those who were previously able to. It is considered abnormal in those older than five years and must be present for at least three months. Like any of the parasomnia group (sleepwalking, sleep eating, etc.), enuresis can be found in any sleep disorder that fragments sleep, such as sleep apnea, but it can also occur in cases of a urinary tract infection (UTI) or congestive heart failure.

Benign prostatic hyperplasia (BPH), also known as benign prostatic enlargement (BPE), is a noncancerous condition that often happens as men age. Their prostate glands become enlarged, and the flow of urine becomes blocked or impeded, which makes it difficult to fully empty the bladder. This may translate into many trips to the bathroom and difficulty sleeping.

Benzodiazepine medications, often referred to as "benzos," are a class of medications that target the benzodiazepine receptors in the brain. They help reduce sleep-inducing antianxiety and have muscle-relaxant properties. The roster includes Xanax (alprazolam), Klonopin (clonazepam), Ativan (lorazepam), Halcion (triazolam), and Valium (diazepam). While they are sometimes prescribed for insomnia and other conditions (see "REM behavior disorder [RBD]" and "Restless legs syndrome [RLS]"), we have to be careful, as they can worsen sleep apnea and be addictive.

The "Big Three" of bad sleep are mentioned throughout this book, but I want to present them as a group because they are so important. The Big Three, as I call them, are alcohol, nicotine, and caffeine. While alcohol and caffeine are typically fine in moderation, nicotine is not. All three can impact sleep negatively, especially when used close to bedtime.

Binaural beats. A newer potential treatment to help with sleep is the idea of binaural beats, which are essentially auditory illusions that are perceived when two different tones are presented through each ear. The listener perceives the auditory illusion of a third tone, in addition to the two pure tones. This third tone is called a binaural beat, which causes the brainwaves to pulsate in sync with the frequency difference. These can be adjusted so the frequency difference will fall into one of the frequency bands, which are known to be associated with specific states of brain activity, ranging from excitement to deep sleep. Some studies have shown that binaural beats can lead to reduced stress, reduced anxiety, increased focus, and increased concentration, to name a few.

BiPAP S/T, which stands for bi-level positive airway pressure spontaneous/timed therapy, is delivered by special BPAP machines (see "BPAP") that are triggered to produce a pressurized breath, either spontaneously (the patient does it) or at fixed time intervals, depending on the settings. While the therapy is quite complicated, the S/T machines assist with impaired breathing, and they can be very useful for patients with central sleep apnea or mixed sleep apnea (combinations of both obstructive and central apnea). They are also used for respiratory insufficiencies, restrictive lung disorders, severe COPD, and hypoventilation syndromes.

Bipolar disorder, which has been called manic depression in the past, is a mood disorder characterized by periods of depression ("down"), followed by periods of abnormally elevated happiness ("up"), and vice versa. Each period can last from days to weeks. If the person becomes psychotic during their "up" phase, it is called mania; if it is less severe, it is called hypomania. In either case, during these periods, the person feels abnormally energetic, happy, irritable, or impulsive, and there is a reduced need for sleep. During periods of depression, the person will need more sleep and will have low mood, low energy, and all the other typical features—conditions that require a psychiatrist. I mention it here because if someone suffers from bipolar depression and they are utilizing cognitive behavioral therapy for insomnia, we must be careful with the use of sleep restriction. Any situation where there is reduced sleep can cause a manic episode to occur.

Blue light. The light that comes from TV sets, smartphones, iPads, computers, LEDs, and fluorescent light bulbs appears to be white but may, in fact, have a frequency in the blue range. This is not good for sleep, because blue light prevents the release of melatonin in the brain, a hormone that makes us sleepy. Turning off these lights and devices at least thirty to sixty minutes before bedtime allows melatonin to be released, making it easier to fall asleep. If I had one tip to impart to our current society it would be this: shut off all screens before bed.

Body temperature. The hypothalamus, which is a structure in the brain, controls many things we don't usually think about, among them hunger and temperature. Body temperature normally drops in the middle of the night. We advise people to sleep in a cooler room for this reason, as the coolness promotes deeper sleep. If you work night shifts or wake up in the middle of the night, you may feel cold, and that is due to the temperature drop that is ingrained in our brains.

BPAP, which stands for bi-level positive airway pressure and is sometimes listed by its brand name, BiPAP, is a medical device that blows pressurized air (not oxygen, just air) into the patient's nose or both the nose and mouth during sleep. Unlike CPAP, BPAP uses two different levels or settings of pressurized air (a higher one and a lower one). The reason for this is to not only keep an airway open (as CPAP does) but also to improve the ability of the lungs to take in oxygen and expel carbon dioxide. The two levels allow for more efficient lung function. The BPAP is also useful in a range of sleep disorders, including obstructive sleep apnea, central sleep apnea, and hypoventilation or hypoxemia in sleep.

BiPAP S/T, which stands for bi-level positive airway pressure spontaneous/timed therapy, is delivered by special BPAP machines (see "BPAP") that are triggered to produce a pressurized breath, either spontaneously (the patient does it) or at fixed time intervals, depending on the settings. While the therapy is quite complicated, the S/T machines assist with impaired breathing, and they can be very useful for patients with central sleep apnea or mixed sleep apnea (combinations of both obstructive and central apnea). They are also used for respiratory insufficiencies, restrictive lung disorders, severe COPD, and hypoventilation syndromes.

Brain fog, a common term in the world of sleep and neurology, is also very nonspecific. Essentially, it refers to symptoms that can affect the ability to think. Patients with brain fog report feeling confused, disorganized, unable to focus, or unable to put thoughts into words. Many medical conditions can lead to brain fog, including pregnancy, multiple sclerosis, cancer, cancer treatment (so-called chemo brain), menopause, and lupus. For the purposes of this book, we will focus on the link between brain fog and chronic fatigue syndrome, depression, medications, and sleep itself.

Many types of sleep medication, including over the counter and prescribed, may result in daytime symptoms such as dizziness, feeling "hungover," or brain fog. Sometimes, taking a medication the first few times may lead to brain fog. Once the brain adjusts to it, these symptoms disappear. This is important to discuss with the prescribing clinician.

Chronic fatigue syndrome, a not very well understood condition, involves tiredness in both body and mind. As with all causes of brain fog, there may be confusion, forgetfulness, and an inability to focus. While there is no cure, many of the remedies mentioned in this book—such as certain medications, regular exercise, and therapy—may be of help.

When people are suffering with depression, brain fog may look like difficulty remembering things or trouble with problem solving, which could be linked to the loss of energy and motivation that comes with depression. It could also be another potential effect of depression on the brain, such as its effect on sleep. Treatment for depression, which includes medication and talk therapy, should also help brain fog.

Proper sleep helps your brain work the right way. However, as is often the case, too much of a good thing can result in feeling foggy the next day. I often see this in major depression, where patients will oversleep, leading to brain fog the next day. The average person needs seven to nine hours of sleep, and while this is not the same for everyone, it is a good place to start. Doing all the things you'll read about through this book (reducing caffeine and alcohol in the evening, keeping a consistent schedule, etc.) will also help, but there may be other issues that should be evaluated. For example, brain fog can be seen in various sleep disorders like sleep apnea, insomnia, and narcolepsy.

Brain injury and sleep disorders. Sleep disturbances often occur with any kind of brain injury, whether it be a stroke (sleep apnea is very common) or from something like a traumatic brain injury. Insomnia, fatigue, and sleepiness are often noted following a concussion. In severe head trauma, narcolepsy can occur, among other issues like sleep apnea. Depression, anxiety, and pain are also common in brain-injury patients and affect sleep quality. In many cases, a sleep test might be a helpful tool to look for sleep apnea or leg kicking through the night (see "PLMS—periodic limb movements of sleep"); treating the underlying problems (whether it be with CPAP, medication, or something else) may help. An injured brain is most in need of good quality and quantity of sleep, so treating any underlying sleep disorder becomes even more important.

Cataplexy is a sudden and short-lived episode of muscle weakness triggered by strong emotions such as laughing, crying, or terror. It is seen only in patients with narcolepsy and is actually diagnostic of the condition.

In patients with narcolepsy type 1, there is a loss of a hormone called orexin (or hypocretin), which helps to stabilize sleep and wakefulness. When it is missing, sleep and wake tend to intrude on one another, and cataplexy is a form of this intrusion. Think of it this way: the loss of muscle strength that people get during normal REM sleep is happening in wakefulness in response to an emotional trigger.

This can appear very dramatically with patients falling to the ground, or, more commonly, it can be something as simple as an inability to keep their head up or being unable to hold a cup during an attack. This condition separates itself from other forms of spells, such as seizures or fainting, in that there is no loss of consciousness; also, after one to two minutes, the patient is usually back to normal.

Fortunately, the medications we use to treat the sleepiness of narcolepsy usually also help with cataplexy. And it is important to note that if you have cataplexy, taking precautions not to put yourself in potentially dangerous situations is absolutely needed (e.g., not standing near the edge on a subway platform).

Catathrenia (nighttime groaning). This is a rare condition in which the patient will groan or moan loudly in their sleep as they exhale. The groaning or moaning sounds last between seconds to nearly a minute, and they typically occur during rapid eye movement (REM) sleep. This condition, which may be very distressing to a bed partner, can be diagnosed during an overnight polysomnogram (PSG). Catathrenia can be treated with continuous positive airway pressure (CPAP).

CBT-I—Cognitive behavioral therapy for insomnia. A collection of behavioral practices used by clinicians to help retrain the brain, CBT-I has been shown to be the most effective long-term way of battling chronic insomnia. We usually combine CBT-I with medication for even more benefit, with the idea of withdrawing the medication after sleep has improved. CBT-I is usually done under the guidance of a cognitive behavioral therapist, but recently several self-help internet programs have come on the market. Regardless of how CBT-I is done, you should always tell your doctors that you are implementing it. The two most important components of CBT-I are sleep restriction therapy and stimulus control therapy, both of which are covered separately in detail in this book.

Central sleep apnea (CSA) is a sleep-related breathing disorder in which the patient essentially stops having the drive to breathe while sleeping. This is different from obstructive sleep apnea (OSA) in that the OSA patient is struggling to breathe against a closed or obstructed airway; in CSA, the stoppages of breathing are usually caused by a faulty or unstable feedback mechanism controlling respiration.

In a normal situation, breathing maintains oxygen and carbon dioxide levels (we breathe oxygen in and get rid of carbon dioxide). Any sudden drop in oxygen or excess of carbon dioxide causes the brain's respiratory centers to breathe.

When someone has CSA, the mechanism is imbalanced during sleep and fails to give the signal to inhale; then the feedback system notices that carbon dioxide is getting high and, in turn, causes the person to breathe quickly and deeply. There is no effort made to breathe during the pause in breathing: there are no chest movements and no muscular struggling, although when awakening occurs in the middle of a pause, it can lead to a feeling of panic.

How do we treat this? That depends on what is causing it: in some cases, CSA is due to the use of opioid medications; in many cases, it is due to congestive heart failure (CHF), but other times, we just don't know. The first step if someone is on an opioid medication is to take them off where possible; if CHF is present, the plan would be to treat that.

Recently, a new implantable device has been introduced, which is similar to hypoglossal nerve stimulators but with a different way of working. Called the Remede system, it is implanted like a pacemaker (see "Remede"). Once in the body, it sends a signal to the phrenic nerve, which is in the chest, to tell the diaphragm to take a breath. Other options include PAP, CPAP, or BPAP (see entries for "Continuous positive airway pressure [CPAP]" and "BPAP"), but it is important to know that both CPAP and BPAP devices can also trigger CSA. In that case, ASV can be used (see *"ASV [adaptive servo-ventilation]"*), assuming the person does not have a severe case of CHF.

One last item to mention here is a condition often seen in patients with CSA that is called "Cheyne-Stokes respiration" (see "Cheyne-Stokes respiration").

This is very confusing, to be sure, but the important things to know are that CSA is different than OSA, has different causes, and that the treatment may be different. However, the results of *not* treating can be the same—cardiovascular problems, feeling exhausted, and other health problems, to name a few.

Cheyne-Stokes respiration. This is a rare, abnormal breathing pattern that can occur while awake, but it usually occurs during sleep. The pattern involves a period of fast, shallow breathing followed by slow, heavier breathing and/or moments without any breath at all (which you'll recall from the entry above is essentially central sleep apnea). After a cycle of fast breathing followed by shallow/no breathing, another begins—typically lasting forty-five to ninety seconds.

The most common causes of Cheyne-Stokes respiration are congestive heart failure (CHF) and stroke. Although considered to be rare, Cheyne-Stokes breathing occurs in 25 percent to 50 percent of people with CHF. But regardless of the cause, it is important to treat Cheyne-Stokes respiration because, like all forms of abnormal breathing in sleep, there can be negative consequences down the road.

Typically, this is managed by treating the underlying problem, which is CHF in most cases. In other cases, oxygen therapy and/or continuous positive airway pressure (CPAP) can be used.

Chronic fatigue syndrome (CFS) is a complex, long-term medical condition which is still not well understood. The core symptoms include flare ups after ordinary, minor physical or mental activity, sleep disturbances, and overall reduced levels of daytime function. Some have proposed the reasons for this condition include biological, genetic, infectious, physical, or psychological stress that affects the biochemistry of the body; sadly, there is no blood test or other lab test to make the diagnosis and show what is wrong.

Fatigue is a common symptom in many illnesses, but the unexplained level of fatigue and the severity of functional impairment in CFS are relatively rare in these other illnesses. Patients may recover from CFS or improve over time, but some don't, and there are no approved treatments for curing the illness. In other words, we can only manage symptoms. It is reported that about 1 percent of primary care patients have CFS. It occurs 1.5–2 times as often in women as in men, commonly affecting adults between ages forty to sixty.

In a sleep specialist's office, fatigue is a somewhat regular occurrence, but unfortunately, there is not a lot we can do. Typically, we will examine the patient, testing for narcolepsy (see entries for "Polysomnography" and "Multiple sleep latency test [MSLT]"). We may do blood work (looking for anemia, low vitamin levels, or low levels of testosterone, the male sex hormone that plays a role in reproduction, growth, and healthy body maintenance), but typically we will not find anything "wrong." In that case, the next step usually involves improving the quality of sleep and/or medications to provide a daytime boost. The good news is that the field of neuro-immunology, which concerns itself with conditions such as CFS, is rapidly expanding. Ideally, in time and with more research, we will have a better understanding of this disabling condition and how to treat it.

Chronic insomnia. "The patient should wake during the day and sleep during the night. . . . The worst part is to get no sleep either night or day, for it follows from this symptom that the insomnolency is connected with sorrow and pains, or that is about to become delirious" (Hippocrates, famous ancient Greek physician, for whom the Hippocratic oath is named).

The term *insomnia* means a person cannot get to sleep, cannot stay asleep, or has unrefreshing sleep (or a combination). It can be extremely distressing both in its acute and chronic types. Here we will talk about the more sinister form, which is chronic and the reason many of my patients come to see me.

Chronic insomnia is, by definition, insomnia that occurs at least three nights per week over a period of at least three months. The best way to understand chronic insomnia is through the "3P" idea put forth by my late colleague, Dr. Arthur Spielman. The first *P* stands for *predisposing*, which refers to a family history of insomnia or a personal history of anxiety or panic, which normally lies just under the surface. The second *P* is for *precipitating*, which could be a divorce, a death in the family, or a job change—any of which leads the predisposing factors to rear their ugly head, and the result is the person will have trouble sleeping. The third *P* is for *perpetuating*, which includes things like bad sleep habits, spending too much time in bed, and seeing bed as a place of stress rather than a place of sleep—all of which keep the insomnia going. The third *P* is where sleep clinicians do their work.

This means helping patients to clean up their sleep habits. As you will see elsewhere in this book, things like improving sleep hygiene, use of sleep restriction, and use of stimulus control therapy are all parts of improving behaviors around the sleep period (see "CBT-I— Cognitive behavioral therapy for insomnia"). Relaxation techniques are also helpful, including mindfulness meditation, hypnotherapy, and acupuncture, all of which can be good to experiment with. I always tell my patients, "If it doesn't hurt, it's worth a try."

In some people, a vicious cycle of insomnia and bedtime anxiety exists. We think of it as a type of performance anxiety in which the very nature of having insomnia makes people anxious about bedtime, which worsens the insomnia. That, in turn, worsens the anxiety, and thus treating both the anxiety and stress in conjunction with the insomnia is of paramount importance. I have seen many cases where patients want the insomnia treated but don't pay enough attention to the anxiety/stress/ depression/ruminating thoughts that are driving it.

In other words, we need to take care of all relevant factors. Yoga, meditation, acupuncture, Tai Chi, massage therapy, and others can be useful. These natural/homeopathic approaches tend to be underutilized for insomnia, which is a shame because they have no side effects and can be incredibly helpful. Additionally, seeing a therapist or psychiatrist can also be very helpful and is something I recommend to many patients.

One thing to note when we talk about chronic insomnia is that sleep is not something that we can "perfect." Some people will never have the full eight continuous hours that we are led to believe is ideal, and this is okay. What we should be looking at is how we can improve the problem (insofar as our habits, etc.) and focus on how we feel throughout the day.

A potential cause of chronic insomnia, one that does not have a root in anxiety, is idiopathic insomnia. While it is often true that insomnia occurs following a major life event, some people have insomnia starting at a very young age. The term *idiopathic* (as with idiopathic hypersomnia) means we do not know why it happens, and, unfortunately, it can be quite difficult to treat.

Regarding treatment, I sometimes see myself as a coach in the sense that I encourage patients to stick with the plan, even if there are bad nights—and to remember that chronic insomnia may have a waxing and waning nature. That said, let's look at some of the things we focus on:

- *Noise:* People who sleep lightly and have difficulty falling asleep may be bothered by even light noise. A white noise machine, a fan, or earplugs may be useful.
- *Substances:* Caffeine, nicotine, and alcohol affect sleep—the Big Three, as I call them (see below). Diet may also impact sleep in that heavy meals close to bed can lead to sleep disruption. A good diet, along with other healthy lifestyle choices, can be beneficial to overall wellbeing. Similarly, diet pills are usually stimulants and can make it difficult to fall asleep at night, especially when taken late in the day.
- *Habits:* Going to bed only when sleepy is a wonderful tactic that people with insomnia tend not to do. Rather, hoping to get more sleep, they often get into bed when they are not sleepy. This leads to lying in bed wide awake with ruminating thoughts, frustration, and anxiety, all of which perpetuate the insomnia. Going to bed only when sleepy, even when it is later in the night, can be a helpful sleep hygiene technique. Some clinicians employ a sleep hygiene technique known as paradoxical intention. This is when we tell patients to say to themselves, "I want to stay awake, I want to stay awake, I want to stay awake . . ."—which usually

has the opposite effect. It helps them sleep by reducing the performance anxiety that comes with being anxious about insomnia and falling asleep.

- *Medications:* Multiple medications and over-the-counter substances can affect sleep. The list is too long to mention, but some to consider are certain blood pressure pills, some anti-depressants, stimulant and wake-promoting agents, and others. Check with your doctor.
- *Outlook:* Having a positive outlook about the bed and sleep environment can have a big impact on sleep. This is important in the reconditioning plan of improving sleep hygiene. Much of the time, insomnia results from the brain having been conditioned to think of bed as a place of stress or anxiety.

Treating chronic insomnia can be done effectively with a combination of improved sleep hygiene, cognitive behavioral therapy for insomnia (CBT-I), and/or medications or over-the-counter substances like melatonin—each of which has its own entries through this book. The literature shows that while medications may have the best track record on a short-term basis, behavioral modification wins out over the long term. A combination approach is probably most effective overall.

I would like to end this section with a look at other things to consider when it comes to chronic insomnia. For example, OSA can lead to awakenings through the night, as can prostate issues in men or hormonal changes in women. On another front, I can't tell you how important anxiety and depression are when it comes to insomnia. Classically, anxiety may cause problems falling asleep, and depression often causes early morning awakening. In many cases, an evaluation by a therapist or a psychiatrist would be helpful.

Certain substances may cause or worsen insomnia; in particular, caffeine, alcohol, and nicotine. Nicotine is a stimulant, which means smoking even a couple hours before bed can lead to difficulty with sleep. Similarly, caffeine can last a while in the body (even hours after the energy boost wears off) and can therefore make it more difficult to fall asleep. In this case, I would recommend people avoid even decaf products, as these have caffeine in them; if there is any trouble sleeping at night, I would suggest only caffeine-free products after twelve o'clock to one o'clock in the afternoon or so.

Finally, people will frequently tell me that a glass of wine with dinner or right before bed helps them sleep. What's interesting is that after falling asleep with alcohol in the system, the first hour or so will usually be okay. But alcohol is a depressant and, once it is metabolized, the body responds in a reverse way. In other words, one may go from being in a relaxed state to suddenly waking up, sweating, with a dry mouth or needing to urinate. Furthermore, it can worsen snoring and OSA, which also leads to awakenings through the night.

Chronic obstructive pulmonary disease (COPD) is a type of progressive lung disease that results from airflow limitation. While OSA is due to obstruction by the tongue, COPD is caused by issues with the lungs themselves. Symptoms tend to be shortness of breath and a chronic cough, both of which get worse over time, increasing the difficulty of everyday activities such as walking or dressing.

The most common cause of COPD is tobacco smoking, but other risk factors include pollution, exposure to occupational substances such as cadmium dust or fumes, and family history. In some cases, there can be what is called overlap syndrome, which is the combination of obstructive sleep apnea (OSA) with COPD. In these cases, oxygen drops further than it would in either case, which can then lead to further heart and lung disease.

Treatment of COPD itself comes in the form of bronchodilators, steroids, and, sometimes, oxygen. With overlap syndrome, the treatment of COPD is combined with the treatment of OSA; continuous positive airway pressure (CPAP) or similar types of devices are needed and are sometimes combined with oxygen. We try to avoid using auto PAP (APAP) in COPD, as these devices can sometimes cause an unsafe increase in pressure in the lungs themselves.

Chronic sleep deprivation has many causes. It also has many unpleasant effects, ranging from tiredness in the morning hours, to mental slowness and prolonged feelings of tiredness throughout the day. Another common result is often a reluctance to engage in physical work or exercise. Reaction time, judgment, vigilance, and overall decision making may be affected by chronic sleep deprivation, and the person may not even be aware of this. Bottom line: we get one hour less sleep than we did one hundred years ago. This doesn't seem like a big deal, but it absolutely can be. Sleep deprivation, if it is chronic, affects long term health, including cardiovascular and neurologic, and may be linked to neurodegenerative illness, like Alzheimer's disease.

Circadian rhythm is a natural, internal process that regulates the sleep–wake cycle and repeats roughly every twenty-four hours. It can be seen in plants, animals and, of course, humans. The term comes from the Latin *circa*, meaning "approximately," and *diēm*, meaning "day." It is important for us to recognize that our circadian rhythms are adjusted to our environment by cues called zeitgebers (German for "time givers"), which include light, temperature, and the like. Light, being the most important zeitgeber, is one of the reasons we should avoid blue light devices (see "Blue light") around bedtime, as this can throw our rhythm off and impact sleeping.

Circadian rhythm sleep disorders (CRSD) are a group of disorders that result in an abnormal pattern of sleeping and waking. They are either due to a problem with one's internal clock or to external factors (such as the use of blue light devices)—or both. In many cases, there is a family history. The conditions include delayed sleep phase disorder (see "Delayed sleep phase disorder [DSPD]"), in which the clock is set "too late;" advanced sleep phase disorder (see "Advanced sleep phase disorder"), in which the clock is set "too early;" and non-twenty-four-hour sleep-wake disorder and irregular sleep-wake rhythm disorder, which are more varied as their names suggest. Treatment of these conditions involves use of bright light at specific times of the day and/or the use of melatonin. Consistency is very important in treating these conditions, particularly irregular sleep-wake rhythm disorder.

Clock watching. Some patients with chronic insomnia can tell us exactly what time they wake every night—the reason: They are clock watchers, which hurts their ability to sleep. It tends to be an issue with those who are overly concerned that they are not getting enough sleep. If these patients do not fall asleep quickly, they check to see how long they have been in bed—or, if they wake in the middle of the night, they may check to see what time it is and calculate how much longer they have to sleep before the alarm goes off.

Unfortunately, these behaviors create anxiety, which only increases their inability to fall asleep. As part of improved sleep hygiene/habits (see "Sleep hygiene") and cognitive behavioral therapy for insomnia (see "CBT-I—Cognitive behavioral therapy for insomnia"), it would be better if patients who feel they have been lying in bed for a long time (usually twenty minutes or so) to get up and go to another room until they feel tired and then get back into bed. They can meditate, read a book, or listen to soft music or a podcast while they get tired and relaxed, but checking the time may work against them.

Compression stockings are specially made, snug fitting, stretchy socks that gently squeeze your legs; they can reduce swelling in your feet and ankles as well as help prevent and treat spider and varicose veins. They are a potential complementary treatment for restless legs syndrome (see "Restless legs syndrome [RLS]").

Confusional arousal is a condition during which an individual experiences a partial awakening from sleep (an arousal) and remains in a confused state. The person will usually remain in bed, sit up and look around, and then return to sleep. The condition lasts anywhere from seconds to minutes. As with most conditions of this nature, by itself it is benign, but the thing I look for is whether there may be another sleep disorder that is triggering it. Just like sleepwalking, it can be common in kids but less so in adults.

Continuous positive airway pressure (CPAP), a device that is usually referred to by its initials, is worn when asleep for the treatment of obstructive sleep apnea. CPAP works by sending pressurized air through either the nasal passages alone or through the nasal passages and mouth, down to the back of the throat. Basically, it acts as an airway split to prevent the tongue and the soft tissues from falling backward and blocking the airway.

There are three main types of CPAP interfaces: the full-face mask (which covers nose and mouth), the nasal mask (covering just the nose), and nasal pillows (plugs that sit in the nostrils themselves). The choice of mask is based on several factors: comfort and size are the big ones, but, if a patient is strictly a mouth breather with a constantly stuffed nose, a nasal interface may not be effective. In those cases, we will opt for a full-face mask. New types of CPAP interfaces come to market every year or so. If you were to talk to someone who tried CPAP twenty years ago, they typically might say something like, "I had a huge Darth Vader thing on my face, and it was horrible." These days we have much smaller interfaces. Even if someone tried CPAP in the past but couldn't tolerate it or didn't want to continue, that is not to say we can't make it work today.

In this day and age, with the field moving ahead rapidly, new masks and equipment are being designed and refined regularly. CPAP can be worth a retry by those who have been initially disappointed. The bottom line is that CPAP does work, and a large amount of medical literature shows how effective it is.

Chronic snoring and OSA produce inflammation of the upper airway. Inflammation results in swelling of soft tissues (similar to what happens in a sprained ankle), and the airway is further tightened as a result of this swelling. Adding CPAP to the mix reduces the inflammation. As a result, in the case of someone who uses CPAP nightly but then stops for a night, the bed partner may say the bed partner is not snoring anymore. While this is correct, it does not mean that the OSA has been cured. Rather, a few more nights without CPAP will often result in the inflammation returning, and the OSA will revert back to where it started, snoring and all. Some people think they will become "addicted" or habituated to the CPAP, which is not correct. They ask, "Will my OSA become worse if I use the CPAP and then stop?" The answer is no, it will go back to what it was before treatment.

People who try CPAP for the first time often have the same complaint: it's uncomfortable, causes claustrophobia, and is noisy, all of which are completely valid. Sometimes it takes extra effort on the part of the provider—as well as the home care medical company that supplies the actual equipment—to work with the patient to get the right mask/pressure setting. In some cases, I will ask patients to add melatonin to their prescribed medications as they adjust to life with the CPAP. This can get them over the hump and increase satisfaction with CPAP in time.

COVID-19 and sleep. In late December of 2019, a new respiratory virus began to spread across the world, called "2019 novel coronavirus (2019-nCoV/SARS-CoV-2)." On January 30, 2020, the World Health Organization (WHO) declared COVID-19 a public health emergency of international concern, and, on March 11, 2020, a pandemic. COVID-19, Omicron and other variants have since infected millions of people worldwide and led to countless deaths. As of the writing of this book, COVID-19 is still a major problem, although thankfully decreasing in the United States.

It is well-known that outbreaks of infectious diseases, along with the measures to control the outbreaks, result in psychologic distress and symptoms, which—not surprisingly—include poor sleep quality. In one study looking at UK households, it was shown that one month after the WHO declared the pandemic, the percentage of adults with mental health problems increased from approximately 23 percent in 2017–2019, to approximately 37 percent in late April 2020, especially in young adults and females. By recent estimates, about one-third of all populations had sleep problems during this time. Patients with COVID-19 appeared to be the most affected group, with as many as 75 percent reporting sleep issues.

As you have seen already, sleep is essential when facing COVID-19 because of its many benefits for mental and physical health. The lack of sleep can impair physical functioning and decision making, lessen the body's immune system, increase accidents, lead to mood changes, make it more difficult to manage anxiety and depression, and even possibly increase the susceptibility to contracting the virus.

To improve sleep quality during these times, people need social and administrative support, the use of relaxation techniques, and reasonable working schedules—all are important to allow for recovery. Seeing a sleep specialist and, of course, following the guidelines in this book are not bad ideas either.

Daylight saving time (DST). During daylight saving time, clocks are turned forward an hour, effectively shifting an hour of daylight from the morning to the evening. As this book was being written, most of the United States began DST at 2:00 a.m. on the second Sunday in March and reverted to standard time on the first Sunday in November. Even though DST gives us the opportunity to enjoy sunny summer evenings by moving our clocks an hour forward in the spring, its implementation has always been the subject of great controversy. Fortunately, in 2022, the US Senate passed a bill called the Sunshine Protection Act, which makes daylight saving time permanent starting in November of 2023.

Delayed sleep phase disorder (DSPD) is a circadian rhythm disorder in which the time a person gets to sleep is delayed by hours beyond the conventional bedtime, which often causes difficulty waking up at the desired time and next-day impairment. While DSPD can be treated by bright light therapy and use of melatonin, a good place to start is to develop and maintain good sleeping habits, which include going to bed and waking up at the same time each day; avoiding caffeinated products and other stimulants like alcohol; maintaining a cool, quiet bedroom; and avoiding smartphone, video games, and other stimulating activities before bedtime.

Delta wave sleep is also known as non-REM stage 3, N3, slow-wave sleep, and, simply, deep sleep. As our brains move through a sleep cycle, they go through the stages of non-REM (see "NREM, or non-REM sleep"): stage N1, then N2, and lastly, N3. In N3, the brainwaves look very distinct, almost like waves on an ocean, demonstrating how the entire brain is in a synchronous, deep state of sleep. Once we are in this very deep sleep state in which we spend about 20–25 percent of our night, it is difficult to wake up from it. Nature has figured that because waking up out of N3 sleep is so difficult, it should be mostly experienced in the first half of the night and less so in the second.

N3 sleep is responsible for sleep inertia (see "Sleep inertia") when it occurs during a nap or when someone is trying to "make up" for lost sleep. In that scenario, to get more bang for the buck, so to speak, the brain will get more N3 sleep at the expense of lighter sleep. As a result, it will occur in the second half of the night or during that nap, thus leading to the possibility of waking up and feeling worse than before falling asleep.

Sleepwalking typically occurs when moving in and out of N3 sleep; thus, the more one gets N3 sleep, the higher chance there is of sleepwalking. This explains why adults who have a predisposition to sleepwalk may have it occur on nights when their sleep schedule has been erratic (the brain trying to make up for what it lost). A better example of this is in children, who tend to have much more N3 sleep than adults, leading to the higher likelihood of sleepwalking as compared to adults.

Dementia is a term used to describe the loss of cognitive functioning, such as thinking, remembering, and reasoning. People with dementia can develop issues with memory, language skills, visual perception, problem solving, self-management, and the ability to focus and pay attention. Dementia can also cause behavioral difficulties that interfere with a person's daily life and activities. There are different forms of dementia, including Alzheimer's disease, Lewy body dementia, frontotemporal disorders, and vascular dementia. While researchers have not come up with a foolproof way to prevent dementia, a good night's sleep is high on most lists.

Depression. After anxiety, depression is the second most common mental health issue in the United States, and it is a major cause of disability worldwide. While we don't know exactly what causes depression, a family history is present in many cases. (Throughout this book, I often use anxiety and depression interchangeably, so please do not let this confuse you. When I use either term, I am referring to *clinical* anxiety/depression, not situational.) I see many patients with depression; sometimes it has been addressed and other times not. It is important to understand that when I say *depression*, I do not necessarily mean the person is walking around with their head down all day, upset because their life circumstances are not what they want them to be. I mean quite the contrary. I am not a psychiatrist, but patients suffering with depression often say that their life is fine, that they have no complaints, and so on, and that their only manifestation of the problem is poor sleep.

In fact, there is a two-way problem when it comes to clinical depression/anxiety and sleep. When a person doesn't sleep well, their mood is affected, and when they have a mood problem, sleep is often poor. In most cases, I find that depressed patients will wake early in the morning or the middle of the night, and they will be tired in the daytime. Sometimes they will sleep all day, and sometimes they will spend all day in bed.

What is confusing for both the patient and the clinician is that these problems can appear to be similar to other sleep disorders. For example, the middle-of-the-night awakening that we see with depression can sometimes look exactly like the middle-of-the-night awakening we see with sleep apnea. Similarly, the daytime sleepiness/fatigue that major depression is known for can look very similar to what we see in conditions of hypersomnia or fatigue (see the entries for "Hypersomnia" and "Fatigue").

We know that insomnia is the most common issue to occur with depression—an estimated 75 percent of people with insomnia have depression. But it is thought that 20 percent of people with depression have sleep apnea and an estimated 15 percent have hypersomnia. You can find more information about that in the entry for hypersomnia, but for now, that simply means being tired. Remember, too, that many people go back and forth between insomnia and hypersomnia during a single period of depression.

In talking about the effect of depression on quality of sleep, some studies have shown a reduction in delta wave sleep (N3 sleep, or slow wave sleep; see "Delta wave sleep"). I consider depression to be one of the two main causes for trouble staying asleep; one is physical problems like sleep apnea (see "OSA—Obstructive sleep apnea") and pain or leg kicks (see "PLMS—periodic limb movements of sleep"), and the other is depression.

I usually tell my patients that anxiety may cause trouble getting to sleep, and depression classically causes problems staying asleep. If someone comes to me and has trouble staying asleep—and other physical causes have been ruled out, like sleep apnea, prostate problems in a man, or hormone changes in a woman—we are sometimes left with the possibility of clinical depression, which is not something to be overlooked or dismissed.

What can be done? Options such as counseling, therapy, and certain types of medications can be a game changer. And since many people with undiagnosed/untreated depression often visit a sleep specialist first, sometimes a referral to a psychiatrist (who can prescribe medications), a psychologist (who works primarily on thoughts/behaviors, etc.), or both can be very helpful. Other techniques such as brain stimulation therapies, including electroconvulsive therapy or transcranial magnetic stimulation, can be useful, and like sleep disorders in general, a combination usually works the best.

As is the case in most sleep disorders, simple things can be helpful. Getting enough sunlight, regular exercise, and meditation practices are all things that I strongly recommend. Finally, it is well known that depression can increase the risk of suicide. The National Suicide Prevention Lifeline, which provides free and confidential support on a twenty-four-seven basis, can be reached at 1-800-273-8255.

Diabetes. The body produces a hormone called insulin, made by the pancreas, which causes the transfer of glucose from the bloodstream to the organs to be used for energy. Glucose is basically sugar. When there is less insulin in the body, or it is not as effective as it should be, the extra sugar in the blood can have severe, long-term consequences. When this happens, it is called diabetes mellitus, commonly known as diabetes.

There are three types of diabetes. In type 1, there is failure of the pancreas to produce enough insulin, caused by an autoimmune response. In type 2, the body's cells fail to respond to insulin properly, commonly caused by a combination of excessive body weight and insufficient exercise. The third type, called gestational diabetes, often occurs in pregnant women and results in sharp increases in blood sugar levels.

More than 450 million people are suffering with diabetes worldwide. Type 2 diabetes makes up about 90 percent of the cases, and rates are similar in women and men. Symptoms often include frequent urination, increased thirst, and increased appetite. Sleep disturbances are closely intertwined with diabetes, especially type 2. It is estimated that one in two people with type 2 diabetes has sleep problems due to unstable blood sugar levels and accompanying diabetes-related symptoms: high blood sugar, which is called hyperglycemia, or low blood sugar, called hypoglycemia. Either can lead to insomnia and next-day fatigue.

Here's how this happens. When the blood sugar is high, the kidneys overcompensate by causing you to urinate more often, which disrupts sleep. Going too many hours without eating or taking the wrong balance of diabetes medication can also lead to low blood sugar at night, which can result in nightmares, breaking out in a sweat, or feeling irritated or confused when you wake up. It goes without saying that having diabetes and taking the medications for it can lead to you feeling fatigued on its own.

As with several of the medical problems we discussed in this book, diabetes and sleep have a two-way relationship. Diabetes not only disrupts sleep, but having poor sleep plays a major role in developing and managing diabetes. Researchers believe that poor sleep may affect blood sugar levels due to its effects on insulin, cortisol, and inflammation. One-quarter of people with diabetes report sleeping less than six hours or more than eight hours a night, either of which can have a negative impact on the way insulin works.

Additionally, it is well-known that when people sleep poorly, it has an impact on two of their hormones—leptin and ghrelin (see "Leptin" and "Ghrelin")— that can lead to seeking relief in foods that raise blood sugar and put them at risk of obesity, which is another risk factor for diabetes. Finally, disturbed sleep or frequent nighttime awakenings can make it more challenging to do the other activities that positively affect health: the big one, of course, is getting enough exercise.

Regarding the long term, we find there is mild evidence to suggest that people with diabetes who do not get enough sleep may be at a higher risk for cognitive problems later in life. The other long-term potential problems that I tend to see as a sleep specialist are sleep apnea (obstructive sleep apnea, OSA) and restless legs syndrome (RLS). There is a lot of information in this book on both problems, but for the purposes of this entry, let me explain briefly how they are related to diabetes.

While OSA does not directly cause diabetes, it is known to increase insulin resistance, even in nondiabetic and nonoverweight people. It also is a very common issue in those with diabetes. In fact, the American Diabetes Association estimates that one-fourth of people with type 2 diabetes also have OSA. Not only does OSA lead to fragmented sleep, it also affects oxygen levels throughout the night which, over time, makes insulin less effective and glucose harder to control. Fortunately, treating OSA with CPAP (See "Continuous positive airway pressure [CPAP]"), especially when combined with exercise, weight loss, and medication, can be effective in helping to manage diabetes. But even before that, it is important to consider the possibility of OSA in someone who has diabetes and snores. In that case, treatment needs to start as soon as possible.

The other condition that we see in diabetes is RLS, which occurs in approximately one in five people with type 2 diabetes. It is marked by tingling or other irritating sensations in the legs that can interfere with getting to sleep. One reason for this is that people with diabetes often have nerve damage due to elevated blood sugar over years. This is called peripheral neuropathy and includes numbness, tingling, and pain in the arms and legs, and it can be a risk for RLS. Either way, evaluation and treatment for diabetes is of the utmost importance in these cases, as well as treating the symptoms themselves.

Diet. A common question that gets brought up in magazine articles I'm asked to write is "What is the best diet to help with sleep?" Until recently, there was not a slam-dunk answer. However, a recent study has shed more light on the subject. Researchers at Columbia University published their findings in an article in the *Journal of Clinical Sleep Medicine* early in 2022, in which they reported that a diet low in fiber and high in saturated fat and sugar is associated with lighter, less restorative sleep with more fragmentation. Thus, adjusting diet to include more fiber and less saturated fat and sugar may be useful in the management of sleep disorders. The research team recommends increasing fruits, vegetables, and whole grains, as well as eating less processed foods—which is not only a good choice for general health, but it can also promote better sleep.

As was discussed in the diabetes entry, when people do not sleep well or long enough, they are setting themselves up for a poor diet with increased fat and sugar. Now we know that this, in turn, will further adversely affect sleep—the very definition of a vicious cycle. While the actual scientific mechanism of how a high-fat, high-carbohydrate diet adversely affects sleep was not measured in this study, the researchers suggested that high-carbohydrate intake delays the circadian rhythm and reduces melatonin secretion, which, as we discuss throughout this book, will lead to falling asleep later.

Another interesting thought from this study is that there could be implications for some dietary-based therapies, such as the high-fat, low-carbohydrate ketogenic diet that has been promoted for several neurologic disorders. Much more research in this field is needed, but for now, I believe we have taken a big first step.

Digeridoo for apnea. The didgeridoo, a wind instrument developed by Aboriginal peoples of Australia at least fifteen hundred years ago, is now used around the world. It is played with continuously vibrating lips while using a special breathing technique called circular breathing (in which the person breathes in through the nose while blowing air out through the mouth).

This instrument has a cylindrical or conical shape. It can be as big as ten feet long but is usually around four feet. Why are we talking about this odd and unique instrument? Because it has been and can be used as an alternative measure to treat OSA.

When we deal with alternative or complementary treatments, it is important to look at the relevant research to show the scientific utility of what we are talking about. The didgeridoo is no exception. A study from 2006 looked at twenty-five patients with moderate OSA. The twenty-five patients were divided randomly into two groups: one set up to get didgeridoo lessons with daily practice and the other, nothing (called the control group), for four months. The patients in the didgeridoo group practiced an average of 5.9 days a week for 25.3 minutes. Compared with the control group, the didgeridoo group experienced daytime sleepiness and OSA improving significantly, and bed partners reported less sleep disturbance.

Is this a reliable method to treat OSA? Perhaps, but much more data is needed. For now, it is best to stick with what we know works. Hopefully in the future, we will have even more options, such as the didgeridoo.

Dopamine is a molecule produced in the central nervous system that is used in several facets of brain and body function. Classically, it is part of the reward system that gives pleasure when a particular action is performed or a particular substance is ingested. It plays a major role in addiction, but it also has a role in sleeping and waking. Medications that enhance the functioning of dopamine receptors are used in both Parkinson's disease and restless legs syndrome/periodic limb movements of sleep. Examples include pramipexole (Mirapex) and ropinirole (Requip).

Dreams. In *Let's Talk About Sleep*, we devoted an entire chapter to dreams. While there is no need to repeat that material, I would like to take a minute to go over the basics.

Spoiler alert: We still don't know exactly why we dream. Some researchers have found that dreams reflect the concerns a person may have in their wakened life, or that dreams themselves are a spiritual phenomenon insofar as being a source of inspiration, but neither has been proven.

We posed the question, "How does dreaming relate to consciousness?" in our first book, but now ask, "What exactly does it mean to be conscious?"

Certainly, one way to look at it is experiencing the world around us, and in dreams, we do just that. In other words, our brains are working overtime during dreams: the idea of taking in all the sensory cues from the environment causes the brain to be fatigued over the course of a day. But in dream sleep—that is, REM sleep—the brain is not only interacting with the environment but is also creating it. In other words, something important must be going on.

A couple of years ago, I wrote an article for the American Academy of Sleep Medicine's newsletter, *MONTAGE*, titled "Proto-consciousness, REM Sleep and How Adam and Eve 'Woke Up.'" In the article, I discussed the idea of dream sleep being a primitive form of consciousness. Sometime in the past, Dr. Allan Hobson, one of the most prominent sleep researchers, coined the term "protoconsciousness," which he saw as a building block to consciousness.

One idea that came out of this is that dream sleep is the groundwork on which the consciousness experience is based. Following up on this idea, dream sleep can be seen as a virtual world model, complete with an imaginary self, moving through a made-up world while also experiencing emotion. Dreams have had religious implications since the beginning of time, and I argued in the *MONTAGE* article that the biblical Adam and Eve were in a dream state until they "woke up" after eating the forbidden apple.

Current scientific and psychological studies have told us a great deal about what goes on when we dream, and in doing so, have opened the door to new and exciting theories. I would like to mention a few here, repeating the caveat that as of right now, we really don't know.

In *The Interpretation of Dreams*, Freud concluded that some part of our psyche is trying to get out or make itself known through dreams—that basically, dreams are ways of wish fulfillment. Any dream can be looked at as a way of getting something you want, in either a literal or symbolic sense.

On the other hand, some have suggested that dreams are simply internally generated patterns of brain activity during REM sleep, and that dream content does not necessarily have any meaning or message for the individual.

Others have put forth the theory that our brain is always storing memories, regardless of whether we're awake or asleep, and that dreams can be a consolidation of memories or that they are based on nonessential information, which is why dreams tend to have bizarre characteristics. In other words, we're essentially filtering out the things that are not important.

Yet another possibility (and my personal favorite) is that dreams prepare us for the stressors of real life. The idea here is that people who experience threatening dreams would be better able to face real threats while awake—presumably, because they've already run through simulations during the night while dreaming. Similarly, another theory suggests that dreams allow us to solve problems, or that dreams allow us to emotionally run through various situations to select the most useful reactions to them.

Finally, the so-called contemporary theory of dreaming puts forth the idea that dreaming is a way for the brain to make connections between an emotion felt in a particular situation and a symbol—a kind of evolutionary coping mechanism that helped our ancestors deal with the life-threatening situations and traumas they experienced more commonly than we do today.

Dreams can also take us in totally unexpected directions. During my research for this book, I discovered that the German chemist August Kekule had a dream that led to a major breakthrough in science. As the story goes, a dream he had in 1890 about a self-devouring snake (the mouth was eating the tail in a circle or ring of sorts) led him to discover that the benzene molecule is composed of six carbon atoms joined in a ring. Benzene is a natural constituent of crude oil and is widely used to make plastics, resins, and rubber. This is another way in which dreams, quite literally in this case, changed the course of science.

It is intriguing to discuss dreams and the theories about them, and science may one day find that using dreams as a therapeutic approach could be an effective way to deal with certain psychological conditions. Either way, the understanding and interpretation of dreams remain one of the last great frontiers for humanity.

Drug-induced sleep endoscopy (DISE). During DISE, patients receive sedation administered by an anesthesiologist in the operating room. As the muscles of the upper airway relax and patients begin to snore and have some blockage of their breathing, the ENT (ear, nose, and throat) doctor will pass a flexible telescope through one side of the nose to evaluate the throat and observe where the potential blockage of breathing occurs in the upper airway. A drug-induced sleep endoscopy is performed to determine whether a patient would be an ideal candidate for surgery—particularly, implanting an Inspire (hypoglossal nerve stimulation) device. It is a minimally invasive, same-day procedure that is well tolerated by most patients and usually takes thirty to sixty minutes.

EEG—Electroencephalogram. A measure of the "brainwaves" we see on a polysomnogram (PSG) sleep study, an EEG is obtained through electrodes that are temporarily glued onto the scalp. These measurements allow us to know, objectively, whether someone is awake and in light sleep, deep sleep, REM sleep, and so on (see "REM sleep" and "NREM, or non-REM sleep"). EEGs are also used to detect seizures, but they require many more scalp electrodes than are used during a PSG.

Electronic devices. I am not opposed to using all electronic devices before bedtime, just the *blue light* ones, such as TV sets, smartphones, tablets, and the like—typically, devices with a backlit display. They are called blue light devices because the screens give off light in the blue range, which tricks our internal clock into believing that sunlight is coming into our eyes.

Elsewhere in this book, I mention that the sun and sunlight are our bodies' most powerful signals to be awake, which they do by shutting off the production of melatonin. Unfortunately, blue light near bedtime can make our brains think that the sun is out and that we should not be falling asleep.

This being the case, one of the key factors in sleep hygiene (see "Sleep hygiene") involves shutting off electronic devices with a backlit screen between thirty and sixty minutes before bedtime. Strides have been made recently to reduce the effects of blue light from electronic devices through the development of special blue-blocking glasses (which have an orange tint) and blue-blocking programs and apps. The best approach, however, would be to just avoid the use of blue light devices before going to bed.

Other electronic devices and applications—such as radios, podcasts, or meditation apps on a smartphone—are fine, so long as your eyes are not staring at the screen. Another question I get is about e-readers. If the screen looks like a piece of paper and you need an external light source, that typically is fine; we want to avoid backlit screens. Using a small lamp or light on a paper or e-reader page is usually okay, so long as it is not too bright and, of course, not shining on your eyes.

EMDR stands for eye-movement desensitization and reprocessing. During EMDR therapy, the patient recalls emotionally disturbing material in brief doses while, at the same time, focusing on an external stimulus. Therapist-directed eye movements are the most common, but there are others such as finger-tapping and audio stimulation. Basically, EMDR is a way of reprogramming the brain to not respond to a stressful event in the way it has been. After a number of sessions, the patient learns that doing something like this on his or her own will help take them out of the moment and relieve stress. This is not hard-core science, but it boils down to the fact that reprogramming the mind can help diminish anxiety, stress, and so on, which can improve sleep.

Epilepsy and nocturnal seizures. When someone has a seizure in their sleep (nocturnal seizures), it is often accompanied by the classic shaking and writhing. It may, however, be more subtle, such as moving the arms or turning the head to one side or another while staying in one position. We call these movements *stereotyped*, in that sufferers may make the same repetitive motions over and over again (like moving the arm or hand). This helps us to distinguish these movements from the movements of other conditions, like confusional arousals, which are much more varied in their behaviors. Additionally, people with nocturnal seizures may wake up feeling very tired.

If there is any possibility of nocturnal seizures or other abnormal movements (such as REM behavior disorder or sleepwalking), an overnight polysomnogram (PSG) sleep test would help the doctor discover what is actually occurring. Some patients tell me their bed partner says that they twitch throughout the night. Involuntary twitching may be a manifestation of seizures when awake, but it may represent many different things when someone is sleeping, including PLMS (see "PLMS—

periodic limb movements of sleep"), parasomnias (see "Parasomnias"), or it may simply be the tossing and turning we see in someone with untreated sleep apnea.

Epilepsy, which is diagnosed in someone who has had more than two seizures or in those having a seizure syndrome (like absence seizures), has another link to sleep besides possible nocturnal seizures: poor sleep quality or quantity may make epilepsy harder to treat, and it may cause a seizure to occur. If someone has untreated sleep apnea and epilepsy, it is imperative to ensure that the sleep apnea gets treated, as well as their using anti-seizure medication.

Epworth sleepiness scale (ESS) is a short questionnaire that asks patients to rate their likelihood of falling asleep during eight common daily activities, such as sitting and reading, watching TV, and riding as a passenger in a car. While not perfect, it does provide a clinician with a sense of how sleepy a person may be.

Estrogen. Hormones play a huge role in our daily lives. Testosterone, estrogen, and progesterone, all of which have effects throughout the human body, definitely affect sleep (see "Progesterone" for specific details). Estrogen is a sex hormone responsible for the development and regulation of the female reproductive system and secondary sex characteristics.

As it relates to sleep, estrogen reduces the likelihood of sleep apnea occurring in women. Once a woman reaches menopause, and estrogen and progesterone are no longer being produced, the airway may be more prone to closure during sleep. What estrogen actually does, among its many effects, is prevent fat tissue from being deposited in and around the throat region. This keeps an otherwise problematic airway wide open until menopause. I have seen many cases where a woman is the exact same weight her entire life, but after menopause, begins snoring and is later diagnosed with sleep apnea. In menopause, hormone changes themselves may lead to insomnia regardless of sleep apnea, and they may require treatment.

Excessive daytime sleepiness is otherwise known as "Hypersomnia." It can be caused by obstructive sleep apnea (OSA), narcolepsy, idiopathic hypersomnia, depression, certain medications or medical diseases, or irregular or inadequate amounts of sleep. While it sounds the same as fatigue, the two are quite different. People with fatigue will not necessarily fall asleep in a meeting or a classroom, but they don't have the energy to do what they want to do. People with excessive day-time sleepiness *will* fall asleep in those circumstances (and in others, including driving). Thankfully, unlike fatigue, there are only few major causes for hypersomnia, and treating them should improve the symptoms. It is usually diagnosed through a combination of an overnight sleep test (polysomnogram or PSG) plus a next-day nap test (MSLT or multiple sleep latency test). We usually deal with this either by treating the underlying problem (in the case of OSA or sleep deprivation) and/or through the use of a stimulant or wake-promoting medications.

Exercise and sleep. Regular exercise helps people fall asleep more quickly and improves the quality of their sleep. I typically recommend that my patients exercise in the morning (or as early as they can), doing cardio for fifteen to twenty minutes. Exercising after work is probably fine, but we don't want to do so too late, as this can potentially activate you and make it harder to fall asleep. I find the combination of early exercise plus meditation at night is a good plan for many people to improve their sleep, regardless of the problem.

Exploding head syndrome is a benign condition that has been described as hearing loud, imagined sounds (like an exploding bomb) when falling asleep or waking up. While the actual causes are not known, theories include the brain not shutting down completely, disrupted sleep, stress, anxiety, or parts of the inner workings of the ear shifting suddenly. If sleep-related issues of this nature (sleep talking, sleepwalking, etc.) occur frequently or are very disruptive, I would consider a sleep test to ensure that we are not missing a trigger like sleep apnea (which, of course, we would treat). Certain types of medications can be used as well, but usually, reassurance is enough.

Fatal familial insomnia (FFI) is an extremely rare genetic disease. It produces extreme sleeplessness, followed by catastrophic symptoms, including death.

To put it simply, genes are blueprints for the proteins in our bodies. When a gene is abnormal, the protein responsible for it will become abnormal as well. In FFI, that protein is abnormally folded. The misfolded protein clumps together and accumulates other misfolded proteins, and the toxic process occurs. As these toxic proteins build, they start killing the cells in the brain where this protein is located, and the brain starts to undergo disastrous changes.

The patient goes from being unable to sleep, to having hallucinations and delirium, to being completely without sleep, and then to death—over a period of about a year and a half. The usual age of onset is about fifty years old. To highlight how rare this is, I want to point out there have only been about twenty-five cases reported in the world in the last one hundred or so years of medical literature.

Unfortunately, there is no effective treatment, and it always results in death. In a way, it's similar to mad cow disease, but that condition develops when a person eats meat that contains an abnormal protein, which then eventually gets to their brain. FFI, by contrast, comes from genetics.

Fatigue is a term for feelings of tiredness that are not necessarily the same as *sleepiness*. They sound the same, but in fact, they are not. People who have excessive daytime sleepiness (see "Excessive daytime sleepiness") will say that regardless of how much sleep they've gotten the night before, they still could take a nap whenever they want. On the other hand, people with fatigue will not report excessive daytime sleepiness; they just don't have the energy to do what they want to do.

While it is possible for someone with a sleep disorder to have both sleepiness and fatigue, the reasons for the two tend to be different, and the distinction is important. Sleepiness is typically caused by sleep apnea, narcolepsy, idiopathic hypersomnia, or from not getting enough sleep in general. The causes of fatigue are more varied and harder to pin down. For example, any of the causes of sleepiness can additionally lead to fatigue, as can conditions like depression, chronic pain, or fibromyalgia (which is also not well understood), vitamin deficiencies, and even some of the foods we eat (gluten, for example).

The food issue and fatigue are covered in detail in my first book, *Let's Talk About Sleep*. I furthermore recommend *Ultra Mind Solution* (2009), written by Dr. Mark Hyman, who also takes a deep look at the subject. In time, I suspect we will have a better understanding of the different causes of fatigue and how to treat them, but for now, all we can do is treat the symptoms and try to think outside the box, looking at stress or diet as possible causes.

Ferritin is the measure of the iron in the body. When a person has restless legs syndrome (RLS) or periodic limb movements of sleep (PLMS), the ferritin level should be checked. According to the Mayo Clinic, normal ranges are 24–336 in men and 11–307 in women. For someone who has RLS or PLMS, we like their level to above the 50–75 range. Iron replacement pills or iron infusion given directly via IV can raise the ferritin level, as can certain foods. Treating the ferritin/iron levels with pills can take months, but once this is accomplished, the symptoms can improve dramatically. Another thing to note is that ferritin can be low in young, menstruating women. But if it is low in older women or men, a further workup typically needs to be done to ensure that there is no bleeding elsewhere. We also may look at the diet, especially in vegetarians, as there may be a deficiency of iron-rich foods.

Fragmented sleep. When someone comes to see a sleep doctor and says that their sleep is fragmented, that they wake up too early or many times through the night, the first question asked would be "Why?"

Difficulty maintaining sleep usually comes from a physical cause or a nonphysical one. A physical cause could be something like prostate issues in a man (to wake to urinate), pain, or possibly another sleep disorder, such as sleep apnea or leg movements (see "PLMS"). A sleep test would definitely demonstrate some of these physical causes. A nonphysical cause would include depression and anxiety. Depression, in fact, is a classic cause of early morning awakening. Typically, in either physical or nonphysical cases, treating the underlying problem should improve the sleep.

Full moon. An interesting subject is how the moon affects sleep. The terms *lunatic* and *lunacy* are older terms based on the observation that on nights with a full moon, there seemed to be an increase in "crazy" behavior.

There is not a lot of medical literature on the subject, but one study from 2013 by researchers in Switzerland is worth mentioning. They examined subjects undergoing overnight sleep tests to see if there were changes on nights with a full moon. The subjects in the study were not aware of the phase of the moon while the study was ongoing. On nights with a full moon, the depth of their sleep was reduced (see "NREM, or non-REM sleep") and less melatonin was produced (see "Melatonin")—both of which would reduce the quality of sleep.

Sleep and behavior/mood are closely tied together, which gives credence to the old adage that on nights with a full moon, people act "crazy." (I hate to use that term. When I say "crazy," I mean "more irritable" or "more anxious.") This being the case, my recommendation is to make sure your sleep is as good as you can make it, so that even on a full moon night, you will do okay.

Gamma aminobutyric acid (GABA) is a naturally occurring neurotransmitter or chemical messenger in the brain. It is sold as a supplement and used for its antianxiety properties to reduce inflammation and chronic pain, as well as to promote relaxation and to potentially improve sleep. Like many of the natural substances (See "Natural substances"), there is not a lot of data on GABA, so be sure to talk with your doctor before starting it.

Gamma hydroxybutyrate is a medication that is used for both narcolepsy and idiopathic hypersomnia (IH), also called sodium oxybate. It is often referred to as the "date rape" drug because it results in very deep sleep and is distributed by only one pharmacy in the United States. Once prescribed, it is taken in liquid form just before bed, essentially allowing patients to get an extra amount of delta wave, or N3 sleep, which is very restorative sleep (See "Delta wave sleep"). The patient wakes up two and a half to four hours later and takes a second dose. This provides another session of very deep sleep, ultimately helping the patient to feel better during the daytime and to deal with some of the other symptoms of narcolepsy—particularly cataplexy.

Side effects usually include nausea or vomiting, dizziness, bed-wetting, sleepwalking, or tremors. The drug cannot be combined with alcohol or other sleeping pills, because it can cause an unsafe reduction in breathing. The brand name Xyrem is approved for use in narcolepsy. The newer version, Xywav, is approved for both narcolepsy and IH. The main difference between these medications is that Xywav has approximately 90 percent less sodium than Xyrem, which equates to the salt in roughly a bag of potato chips. I often tell patients that despite the oddities of this medication, gamma hydroxybutyrate can be very effective and is worth consideration.

Ghrelin is a hormone made by our stomach signaling that we are hungry. When someone has a sleep disorder (like sleep apnea), or their sleep is disrupted or deprived from other reasons, there may be an increase in ghrelin. This has the effect of turning on the "I'm hungry" signal, possibly leading to overeating. In the case of sleep apnea, this overeating can cause weight gain, which would then make the sleep apnea worse. This would be followed by a further ghrelin increase, more weight gain, and so on—a truly vicious cycle. On top of that, in the case of disrupted sleep, the other important hormone, leptin (which gives the "I'm full" signal), is either decreased or less effective (see "Leptin"). This means the "I'm hungry" signal is activated and the "I'm full" signal is shut off, both of which can lead to problems.

Glymphatic system. In 2013, researchers at the University of Rochester made a profound discovery as to why we sleep—they found that during deep sleep, the supporting cells of the brain shrink in size. It is believed that this allows for the flow of fluid, resulting in the removal of waste products. Because the waste products are toxic to nerve cells, deep sleep allows the brain to recover from a day's worth of thinking and doing. Recent data suggest that quality and duration of sleep may predict the onset of Alzheimer's disease and that adequate sleep may reduce its risk. One model of how this is believed to occur is through the buildup of toxins that are not removed, via the glymphatic system, due to chronically poor sleep.

Grief and sleep. When people are experiencing bereavement from having lost a spouse, a child, a relative, or a friend, sleep is going to be negatively affected. Grief and sleep play on each other, and sleep will definitely be affected by grief—especially if psychological problems like depression and anxiety are already present. It's important to have proper treatment either with a psychologist or counselor for counseling and/or a psychiatrist for medication, which may help the grief itself and thus, ideally, keep sleep difficulties at bay.

Gut and sleep. The bacteria in the gastrointestinal system is there to help us break down food; the combination of all the bacteria in the gut is called the gut biome. When we don't sleep well, the gut biome changes, which has consequences in terms of energy level, our ability to digest, and our ability to function in life. When the gut biome changes, our ability to sleep also gets affected. This is a subject of intensive research at the moment.

Heartburn. See "Acid reflux."

Hemoglobin. Our red blood cells transport oxygen to all tissues of the body. Hemoglobin is the molecule in red blood cells that allows for this transport, and its level can be measured through simple blood tests. If your hemoglobin level is lower than normal, it could signal anemia or even certain types of cancers. In cases of sleep apnea or other breathing-related conditions, the hemoglobin blood level may actually be high.

Histamine. Many people have heard of histamine as it relates to diphen-hydramine (Benadryl), which is an antihistamine known to make them sleepy. Histamine, then, is a neurotransmitter in the brain that causes us to be alert and awake. Recently, a new medication has appeared on the market called pitalosant (Wakix), which works on the histamine system to improve sleepiness and cataplexy caused by narcolepsy.

Home sleep testing. Compared to an in-lab polysomnogram (PSG), which consists of an overnight test at a sleep facility and uses many wires and electrodes, a home sleep test simply measures air flow (via a sensor in the nose/mouth), oxygen level (a sensor on the finger), and body position (side vs. back). Although most people tend to find a home test easier to tolerate and more comfortable than an in-lab PSG, home tests do not measure actual sleep time or account for other problems that may occur during sleep. They only look at the possibility of obstructive sleep apnea (OSA).

At this point in time, many insurance carriers will not cover a PSG, at least initially. And for this reason, a home sleep test is needed.

If the test comes back positive (i.e., OSA is found), then treatment can be prescribed. For example, if we find someone has OSA from their home test, we could send an order to a medical supply company to get them started on an auto-adjusting CPAP (APAP). If the home test comes back negative but the person is having symptoms—either of OSA (e.g., snoring or tiredness) or other issues (e.g., leg kicking)—then a PSG would typically be approved.

Homicidal somnabulism, otherwise known as homicidal sleep-walking, describes a terrifying event—one in which an individual awakens to discover that they murdered someone while they were sleeping. Just like regular sleepwalking, they have no memory of the actions that were taken during their slumber.

Sleep medicine experts are sometimes called to testify as to whether a particular murder is a possible sleep-induced phenomenon. The answer is often: yes, it is possible but very difficult to prove. Sleepwalkers are known to do strange things, such as cook, clean, iron, and even drive a car. But sleepwalking accounts for, luckily, very few of the murder cases.

Sleepwalking itself is potentially dangerous, and the possibility that you could hurt yourself or another person is reason enough to take steps to prevent it. Good sleep practices, taking care of any underlying sleep disorder (like sleep apnea), and avoiding substances that can cause sleep-walking (e.g., Ambien and/or alcohol) are paramount.

Hot flashes and night sweats/hormone therapy. Hot flashes are typically experienced as a feeling of intense heat with sweating and a rapid heartbeat, and they generally last from two to thirty minutes. They are often caused by the change in hormone levels that are characteristic of menopause, often occurring as blood vessels narrow and then widen. Severe hot flashes can make it difficult to get a full night's sleep, and night sweats may also be present. In fact, some women get night sweats without having hot flashes during the daytime.

Hormone replacement therapy (HRT) may relieve many of the hot flash symptoms, but that relief comes at possible risk. Oral HRT has been known to increase the risk of breast cancer, stroke, and dementia. Since it has other potentially serious short-term and long-term risks, HRT is worth a discussion with your OB/GYN practitioner.

Women who experience troublesome hot flashes are advised by some to try alternatives to hormonal therapies as the first line of treatment. These include selective serotonin reuptake inhibitors (SSRIs), such as paroxetine (Paxil), clonidine (a blood pressure-lowering medication that can reduce the narrowing and widening of blood vessels), and isoflavones (like in chickpeas). Other substances such as soy, flaxseed, red clover, ginseng, and yams may relieve hot flashes. Acupuncture, one of my favorite treatments, can also be helpful in dealing with hot flashes.

Hypersomnia. See "Excessive daytime sleepiness" and "Idiopathic hypersomnia."

Hypnagogic/hypnopompic hallucinations are either auditory or visual hallucinations that occur as someone is falling asleep (hypnagogic) or waking up (hypnopompic). These classically occur in narcolepsy but can be seen in other conditions, such as obstructive sleep apnea (OSA). Think of it as someone being half asleep (in dream sleep) and half awake, so there is dream imagery in wakefulness. There also may be a frightening sensation of being unable to move (see "Sleep paralysis"). In the medical literature, some theories suggest that people's reports of alien abductions were really sleep hallucinations in conjunction with sleep paralysis. Typically, these are benign, but like many sleep disorders discussed in this book, it is always best to rule out underlying causes of sleep disruption if they happen frequently.

Hypnosis is something that most people have heard of, but they are not sure exactly what it is or how it is done. Someone in a hypnotized state has focused attention and, as a result, reduced awareness of their surroundings, which results in an enhanced capacity to respond to suggestions. How this happens is a matter of debate. Some argue that the person entering an altered state is in a trance of sorts that is different from normal consciousness; others argue that hypnosis as a treatment is a form of placebo effect. Either way, hypnosis can be useful in pain management, smoking cessation, and dieting. As a way to treat and deal with insomnia, hypnosis can have a positive effect. As in the case of acupuncture, however, the American Academy of Sleep Medicine has not listed hypnosis or hypnotherapy as recommended routes to take. But as I always say, if it *may* help and won't hurt, it might be worth a try.

Hypnotics (sleep aids). The medications and substances that help people sleep can be broken down into several categories:

- Benzodiazepine drugs (sometimes referred to as "benzos") include alprazolam (Xanax), clonazepam (Klonopin), lorazepam (Ativan), and diazepam (Valium). These are medications that help the brain and body relax and are not actually sleeping pills per se, but they are more so antianxiety medications; usually they're used in the psychiatric realm to reduce clinical anxiety, panic attacks, and the like.
- The so-called nonbenzodiazepine drugs (the "nonbenzos") like eszopiclone (Lunesta), zolpidem (Ambien), and zaleplon (Sonata), also known as the "Z" drugs, activate the benzodiazepine receptors in the brain without actually being benzodiazepine drugs. They don't relax the muscles or reduce anxiety as much as benzodiazepine drugs, but they do have a sleep-inducing effect.
- Melatonin-based substances, such as over-the-counter melatonin supplement pills or gummies and the prescription medication ramelteon (Rozerem), may be effective in some cases. See "Melatonin" for more information.
- Suvorexant (Belsomra), lemborexant (Dayvigo), and daridorexant (Quviviq) have an entirely different way of working compared to the other drugs mentioned. They basically block the orexin system in in the brain. Orexin is a neurotransmitter that keeps us awake, so by blocking it, these medications may help to induce sleep.
- Multipurpose medications like Lyrica (pregabalin) or Neurontin (gabapentin), which are used for conditions like seizures, headaches, and pain, as well as sleep, basically slow down the nervous system and can lead to sleep.
- Others include antidepressants like trazodone, mirtazapine, and doxepin (Silenor), as well as an antipsychotic like quetiapine (Seroquel), which tend be used off label but can be very effective, especially if anxiety or depression are also present.

- Advil PM, Tylenol PM, and other over-the-counter preparations like Benadryl contain diphendydramine, which is an antihistamine that causes sleepiness.
- Natural preparations like cherry extract, valerian, and a variety of others are used.

There are always risks connected to anything we put into our bodies, and each category has potential problems that should be noted. In all of them, dizziness or feeling hungover the next day are strong possibilities, and this becomes important to consider when they are used in older people who often experience unsteadiness in the middle of the night.

Specifically, with the benzos, there are risks of addiction. With the nonbenzos and the gabapentin/pregabalin groups, there is a possibility that obstructive sleep apnea (OSA) will become worse on the nights they are taken. Gabapentin/pregabalin can also cause weight gain, as can antipsychotics like quetiapine. Most striking, however, is the good portion of the benzos/nonbenzos and even some of the over-the-counter (diphenhydramine) and antidepressant medications that have been linked to memory problems. The bottom line is drugs can become a complicated issue when they are used long term. And even with the natural substances, I strongly advise consulting a doctor before starting any of the over-the-counter or herbal preparations.

Some over-the-counter substances like ibuprofen (Advil), acetaminophen (Tyenol), and others can affect the liver over time. It is not good to take them often if they are not needed. As for the PM versions (Advil PM, Tylenol PM, etc.), they usually contain diphenhydramine or something similar, and while this is okay in the case of a cold or other short-lived problems, I would not recommend them long term, as they can affect memory.

With any of these substances, a major issue that needs to be mentioned is whether other sleep conditions have been properly addressed. For example, if someone has OSA and is waking up in the middle of the night because of stoppages of breathing, a benzo or nonbenzo may not be the best choice. Instead, treating the OSA and seeing the effect it has on the insomnia would be preferable.

Hypoventilation. The term hypoventilation, which is sometimes called respiratory depression, refers to a situation in which the lungs are unable to get rid of the carbon dioxide (CO_2) in the blood. Our normal breathing consists of taking oxygen in and breathing carbon dioxide out. Carbon dioxide is a waste product of our body's metabolism, and it needs to be eliminated with each breath. Trouble getting rid of the carbon dioxide may be caused by several different underlying causes, including neurologic illness (like Lou Gehrig's disease), certain medications or illicit drugs (opiates or benzodiazepine medications when taken in excess), or morbid obesity. In the case of morbid obesity, the excess fat tissue around the chest makes it hard for the lungs to do their job; this is called obesity hypoventilation syndrome.

In the long term, hypoventilation can result in raising blood pressure, cardiac arrhythmias, disorientation, lethargy seizures, unconsciousness, and, eventually, death. One way to treat these problems is a BPAP (see "BPAP"), which helps increase the efficiency of the lungs. When the hypoventilation is due to obesity, losing significant weight (either through diet and exercise or through bariatric surgery, like a gastric sleeve), can be curative.

Hypoxemia. While hypoventilation refers to a problem getting carbon dioxide *out*, hypoxemia refers to an issue of getting oxygen *in*—usually because of a problem with the lungs. A variety of conditions can cause hypoxemia, including chronic obstructive pulmonary disease (COPD, emphysema), severe asthma, obesity, neurologic illness, sleep apnea (both obstructive and central), and very high altitude. Treatment depends on the underlying problem but may include the use of supplemental oxygen from a tank or a concentrator (as in COPD), weight loss (sometimes bariatric surgery), continuous positive airway pressure (CPAP), bi-level positive airway pressure (BPAP), or other forms of ventilation. On some occasions, we will combine the treatments (e.g., CPAP with supplemental oxygen running through it).

J

Idiopathic hypersomnia (IH). Whenever you hear the term *idiopathic* in medicine, it basically means "we don't know why." Hypersomnia is excessive daytime sleepiness. People with idiopathic hypersomnia are sleepy without a clear understanding of why. The brain has neurotransmitters which lets us know when it's time to be awake and time to be asleep. There is some thought that these neurotransmitters are faulty in regards to IH, but there is not a clear understanding just yet.

A recently approved treatment called Xywav has emerged for IH. Gamma hydroxybutyrate, also known as sodium oxybate (Xyrem), is a liquid that people take at nighttime (usually at bedtime and then a few hours later) that helps them get very deep sleep—essentially, giving them more bang for the buck. In other words, if they sleep for eight hours, it's like they slept for ten, and they wake up more refreshed. Xywav is just like Xyrem, except it has 90 percent less sodium (see "Gamma hydroxybutyrate"). This is the only FDA-approved treatment specifically for IH. Other treatments include off-label use of stimulants and wake-promoting agents.

iNAP (Intra-oral negative air pressure). A treatment for obstructive sleep apnea (OSA), called the Winx system, came and went in the last decade. It worked by sucking the soft tissue of the upper airway forward, which is opposed to continuous positive airway pressure (CPAP) that works by blowing pressure into the airway. The sucking feature stabilized the tongue, making the upper airway space larger, and thus (in theory) reducing snoring and OSA. Unfortunately, the Winx system was wrought with problems, including the fact that insurance carriers were not covering it, that there was no way of knowing beforehand whether it would work, and that there was no way to monitor patient improvement or compliance. It was discontinued in 2017.

It was replaced, in a sense, by the iNAP system: a new, battery-operated, negative intra-oral pressure device, which works similarly to Winx in that it sucks the tongue forward, opening the airway. It is approved for adults with all levels of OSA (including severe). Additional features include an app for mobile devices that tracks usage and seal time; the data can be viewed by providers on a secured website and by patients on their smartphones. Like several other options (NasalEPAP, eXciteOSA, etc.), insurance is not yet covering iNAP, and larger, longer-term studies are needed before it can be considered a widespread solution. But it is important that we have options for treating OSA besides CPAP, surgery, and dental devices, so I am hopeful that iNAP sticks around.

Insomnia. Everyone has heard of insomnia, and everyone has experienced it, but what exactly *is* insomnia? Simply put, it is defined as a complaint of difficulty initiating sleep, maintaining sleep, or waking up too early—also, sleep that is chronically nonrestorative or poor in quality. These issues must be present despite adequate opportunity and circumstances for sleep, and it must result in lower quality daytime functioning. In other words, the sleep must be poor even though there is ample opportunity, and it must make the next day less pleasant than it otherwise might be. It is extremely common, especially in women, who report suffering with insomnia about 50 percent more often than men.

There are several types of insomnia. Both acute and chronic forms have their own entries in this book, and I urge interested readers to go there (see "Acute insomnia" and "Chronic insomnia"). Other types include idiopathic insomnia, paradoxical insomnia, and insomnia associated with or due to a medical, psychiatric, or neurologic condition. The last one is self-explanatory, and it is touched on through this book. The bottom line is if you have a medically significant condition, or if you are on medication or using illicit substances or too much alcohol, your sleep is going to be affected. Another thing to mention is that sleep apnea is a major cause of insomnia, and it should never be overlooked.

Idiopathic insomnia is also known as childhood onset insomnia or life-long insomnia. These are, unfortunately, extremely difficult cases to treat. You will run across the term "idiopathic" at another point in this book (see "Idiopathic hypersomnia"). Essentially, it is a term that means "we don't know why," which is frustrating for patients and clinicians alike. We do our best in these cases, but with this form of insomnia, we are limited.

The other form is paradoxical insomnia, which is also called sleep state misperception, subjective insomnia, pseudoinsomnia, or sleep hypochondriasis. Many times, this is seen in people with severe anxiety. What is happening here is that the patients swear they are not sleeping more than one hour or so per night, and they say it has gone on for decades. The reality is that you cannot live with that type of prolonged sleeplessness. To make this clear, we often do a sleep test (in the office) and show the patient that they are in fact asleep when they think they are not. The test itself can be curative.

Regardless of the type of insomnia, the rules for treating it are the same. This is true if there is any medical, psychiatric, or neurologic condition that should be treated, which includes sleep apnea. After that, there has to be a combination of improved sleep habits (see "CBT-I— Cognitive behavioral therapy for insomnia") and, if needed, medication or over-the-counter substances or supplements (like melatonin) are recommended. I also ask patients to get into the habit of doing cardio exercise in the morning and winding down at night (or in the middle of the night if needed) with mindfulness or guided meditation. The specifics of all these treatments can be found throughout this book. Go for it!

Inspire (and similar devices). The hypoglossal nerve has a very specific function: it controls the tongue. In 2014, the US Food and Drug Administration approved an upper airway stimulation system for use in patients with sleep apnea. It works by delivering a mild electrical stimulation to the hypoglossal nerve in order to increase the muscle tone of the tongue, so it will not collapse into the airway during sleep.

The Inspire device is one such product; however, there are several others, including the Genio and Aura 6000 devices. They all have differences in terms of the type of stimulation, monitoring, battery life, and so on, but the underlying principles are the same.

When I describe these devices to patients, I say that it is like a pacemaker that gets implanted into the body by an ear, nose, and throat (ENT) doctor, and it includes a wire that clips onto the hypoglossal nerve. Once it is implanted and the patient is healed from the surgery, the device is calibrated during an overnight sleep test and is ready to go. The patient turns it on with a remote control before bed, and the device does the rest.

Working with the hypoglossal nerve is especially nice in that it does not have a sensory component, so the patient should not feel the impulses. (Some say they feel a mild vibration, but nothing painful.) The other good thing is that there are two of them, which means the danger of damaging the nerve and then being left with a paralyzed tongue is reduced.

I should mention that for anyone to undergo this procedure, which is done by an ENT surgeon, he or she would have to first undergo what is called a drug-induced sleep endoscopy (see "Drug-induced sleep endoscopy [DISE]"). This shows the ENT doctor exactly how the throat closes during sleep and whether the person would be a good candidate for the procedure.

All of this sounds a little strange and far out, but the big question is "does it work?" And the answer is: yes. I typically reserve this for cases where someone has a very severe case of sleep apnea but cannot use the CPAP, despite his or her best efforts. Other sleep and ENT doctors use it in less severe cases as well, but it all depends on the dialogue between patient and clinician.

IPAP and EPAP refer to the transition from breathing inward (inspiratory positive airway pressure) to breathing outward (expiratory positive airway pressure). They are used in relation to certain CPAP-type devices, especially BPAP, EPAP, and IPAP, which are set according to the patient's breathing patterns and range. The term EPAP is also used to describe "nasal EPAP" appliances that fit over the nose and filter nasal breathing, which can be useful in dealing with sleep apnea and snoring (see "Nasal EPAP").

Iron deficiency. Iron is present in all cells in the human body. For the red blood cells, it is a key component of hemoglobin, which allows for the transport of the oxygen we breathe in to get to all the cells of the body. When iron is low, we call this anemia. There can be many causes; the one I am going to focus on here is in young menstruating women.

The blood loss during a woman's period can result in low iron, which in itself can bring on restless legs syndrome (see "Restless legs syndrome [RLS]"). Iron is used in red blood cells, but it also has a function in the creation of dopamine (see "Dopamine"), which is a neurotransmitter made in the brain and that has many functions. It is believed that reduced dopamine caused by reduced iron is a reason for RLS. The way we measure iron stores in the body is through a blood test called ferritin (see "Ferritin").

If the RLS patient is a young woman, the iron deficiency is typically caused by menstruation. If we see this in an older woman or a man, we look for possible causes of bleeding or find out what the diet is like (vegetarians can have this). If ferritin is low, we treat it with over-the-counter iron supplements taken with orange juice (vitamin C helps absorb iron) or prune juice, which also has vitamin C and can offset constipation. It usually takes a few months for the ferritin to come up; once it does, the RLS symptoms may improve a little or even a lot. In severe cases, iron infusions are used. Other symptoms of iron deficiency often include fatigue, dizziness/lightheadedness, hair loss or thinning, twitches, irritability, weakness, or brittle nails.

J

Jet lag, a relatively recent phenomenon in human history, has existed only since the advent of flight travel. The first known use of the term was in 1965. While not really a disorder, it can be unpleasant. As a rule, it takes roughly a day for our bodies to get realigned for every time zone we travel through by plane.

If you travel one time zone away—say, a flight from New York to Chicago—it would take one night for you to get back to your normal circadian rhythm (see "Circadian rhythm"). If you travel to Europe, which is about five or six hours ahead of New York, it may take a week or so before you're adjusted to the new time period. And while you're there, your brain and body may be completely out of sync. You may be tired in the daytime and activated at night, which could have consequences for work, fun, or whatever you're doing.

There are ways to treat jet lag that include utilizing sunlight in the morning and melatonin at night. The traveler would start by taking melatonin at 9:00 p.m. the first night, and then he or she would wake up at 6:00 a.m. and get some sunlight. Night 2: he or she takes melatonin at 8:30 p.m., wakes up at 5:30 a.m., and then gets some sunlight. For sunlight, I recommend that people go outside for roughly twenty minutes, not staring at the sun but just being in the sun (even on a cloudy day). When they get sunlight in the morning, they're shutting off melatonin and telling their body this is the time to be awake. There are also great online resources to further help (see below).

Because of jet lag, you probably shouldn't be doing anything significantly important the first or second day after your flight. Depending on what time you land and what you have planned for the day, it's probably best to hold off if you have an important meeting or to wait at least a few days, so you can be at your best.

Jet Lag Rooster (jetlagrooster.com) is a program that guides you in ways to shift your body clock before and during a plane flight in order to reduce or prevent jet lag. It creates an individual plan suggesting the best times for exposure to bright light (sunlight) and melatonin. Research suggests that shifting your body clock before departing can sometimes prevent jet lag completely. The program is free and recommended by the Center for Disease Control.

K

Kaizen, which comes from Japan, translates into "good change," a concept of making big changes over time using incremental steps. Interestingly, kaizen, which began as a business theory, helped brands like Toyota achieve major success.

The idea of not jumping headfirst into any major change but doing so slowly and deliberately is a great tool for sleep. When I tell a patient it's time to improve their behaviors around sleep, I may give them ten or so things to focus on. This, understandably, can be overwhelming, so I tell them to start with one or two changes and to move on from there.

Kaizen is effective in bringing about positive change because the emphasis is on starting small and making the tiniest change toward the desired end. This helps to shortcut the brain's natural inclination to resist change.

Kicking in the night. See "Restless legs syndrome [RLS]" and "PLMS—periodic limb movements of sleep."

Klein-Levin syndrome is a rare but troubling disorder that may be triggered by a virus, although this is still not entirely clear. It is comprised of three major symptoms: (1) hypersomnia, which means people are very sleepy; (2) hyperphagia, which means they eat excessively; and (3) hypersexuality, which is obvious. The hypersomnia may result in patients sleeping up to twenty hours per day or more. It usually lasts for a few months and then improves, though it may return and have a recurrent pattern throughout life—

or it may never return again. It's extremely rare, occurring in one out of one million people, and it is not well understood. It is also unknown why it primarily affects males. Treatment is usually just supportive. Lithium, which is used for several psychiatric disorders, may help.

Leptin is a hormone made by our adipose tissue, otherwise known as fat cells. It basically gives us the signal that we have had enough to eat. It is the flip side of ghrelin, which is made by our stomachs and tells us we are hungry. When someone has disrupted sleep—such as from sleep apnea—there may be leptin resistance or a decrease in leptin levels. This has the effect of shutting off the "I'm full" signal.

As a result, patients with sleep apnea (or other causes of disrupted sleep) may end up eating more than they need, which may lead to weight gain. This would make sleep apnea and the sleep disruption worse, and this, in turn, would make leptin less effective, leading to more weight gain, and creating a truly vicious cycle. On top of that, in a case of disrupted sleep, ghrelin increases (see "Ghrelin"), which means the "I'm hungry" signal is activated and the "I'm full" signal is shut off—not a good combination.

Lucid dreams occur when you are aware that you're dreaming while you're asleep. In addition, some people may be able to control how the dream unfolds. We don't know exactly how and why lucid dreams happen, but some ideas suggest that the brain is in a kind of half-wake / half-dream state.

Some have suggested that lucid dreams might be of use in daily life for reducing anxiety (e.g., nightmares can be controlled this way) and for increasing creativity (coming up with new ideas or insights). But others have reported that lucid dreaming may result in reduced sleep quality.

While there is no guaranteed way to cause a lucid dream, some studies have shown that people had more of them when they kept a log of their dreams—presumably, because they were more focused on them.

Also, the idea of devices to trigger a lucid dream has been around for decades, and some masks and headbands have sounds or lights that might bring on a lucid state.

Like dreaming in general, there is still a lot to learn about lucid dreaming. Perhaps one day, they will be used as treatment for psychiatric disorders, as one example. Until then, they remain a very interesting topic, not only for clinicians and researchers but for humanity in general.

M

Mandibular advancement device (MAD). This is a mouth guard that sits over both the upper and lower sets of teeth, and it is used to treat snoring and obstructive sleep apnea (OSA). It works by pulling the lower jaw (the mandible) forward a few millimeters, when worn at bedtime. This has the effect of pulling the tongue and soft tissues away from the back of the throat and opening the upper airway. While mouth guards for teeth grinding (bruxism) are very common, MAD is a little different and does more than just protect the teeth, even though it can be used in place of a simple, grinding mouth guard. While a high-quality version of MAD is usually made by a dentist (useful for OSA), a temporary one can be purchased online (useful for snoring). I usually reserve these for patients with mild to moderate OSA or for a severe case where a patient cannot tolerate continuous positive airway pressure. Sometimes, insurances may not cover them, which may end up costing a patient hundreds or even thousands of dollars. But, if it works, it can be a huge benefit.

Marijuana. I am frequently asked about marijuana and marijuana-type products. While some data shows that marijuana can be useful to reduce anxiety and pain, but whether it helps sleep is a matter of debate. As of now, we are unclear about the long-term effects of marijuana on the brain.

It is known that REM sleep is inhibited by marijuana use. Ask anyone who uses marijuana products regularly, and they will tell you that if they ingest them (either through smoke or otherwise) daily and then stop for a time, the dreams they experience will be much more intense, vivid, and even nightmarish at times. What they are experiencing is REM rebound, which is a consequence of chronically suppressing REM sleep.

The big question is, Is it worse for someone with severe anxiety or pain not to sleep at all, or to have sleep that is REM deprived? We don't know the answer, which is why it important for people to check with their doctor before they try marijuana. Just because marijuana is "natural" does not mean it is 100 percent safe. That said, I am convinced that marijuana can have a place in the right context, but only time and rigorous research will give us definitive answers.

Massage therapy. If you have trouble sleeping, I would consider getting a professional massage. The purpose of massage is generally for the treatment of stress, pain, and even sleep. The types of massage are varied, including Swedish, deep tissue, structural integration, trigger point, manual lymphatic drainage, sports massage, Thai massage, and others.

Is massage therapy right for everyone? And what is the best kind for insomnia? I am not sure these questions have been answered or will ever be answered in a definitive way. However, if you have access to someone who performs massage and you have the means to experience it yourself, it is worth checking out. Anecdotally, when I get a massage, it helps me not just to sleep but also in reducing tension and feeling better.

Mattresses. We spend a third of our lives in bed, which makes our choice of mattress an important one.

Fortunately, there are hundreds of different mattresses on the market, dozens of reliable companies that rate them (*Good Housekeeping, U.S. News and World Report*, etc.), many online sites that discuss and describe in detail the various types on the market, and many reputable companies—both retail and online—that not only sell and deliver them but also offer test drives and money-back guarantees if the first ones don't work.

I am often asked which mattress a patient should purchase, and my response is typically centered around two things: the degree of firmness a person requires and technology.

I prefer a firmer mattress for my patients because it facilitates sleeping in the fetal position (on the side) more than the softer mattresses, but I also want it to be comfortable. As *U.S. News and World Report* discusses in its examination of the field, firmness levels range from soft to firm, with a scale from 1 to 10 (the higher numbers signifying a firmer mattress). The most popular mattresses appear to be medium–firm (between 6.5 and 7.5) and firm (8 to 10). For details, see the *U.S. News and World Report* 2022 mattress guide (www.usnews.com/360-reviews/sleep/mattress).

A medium–firm mattress supports the head, neck, and spine, which is critically important. I recommend that people sleep on their side in the fetal position, with their head and neck supported by a pillow and the hips and knees flexed at ninety degrees (with maybe a pillow between the legs for comfort). When a person is on his or her side like that, it puts the body in a neutral position, so everything is in alignment. Sleeping on your side is also good if you suffer from snoring and/or obstructive sleep apnea (OSA)—there is less chance that your airway will become small (leading to snoring), or closed off (leading to OSA) if you are sleeping on your side versus on your back. You want a mattress that can accommodate that.

The two main components of bed technology include temperature factors and antimicrobial materials. While the need for antimicrobial materials might be obvious, the need for temperature regulation may not, but it can make a significant difference in sleep quality. A National Sleep Foundation poll found that a cool room temperature was one of the most important factors in getting a good night's sleep. While it can certainly vary from person to person, the best bedroom temperature for sleep is approximately sixty-five degrees. Our bodies are programmed to experience a slight dip in core temperature in the middle of the night, and if a mattress can assist this process, all the better.

As I mentioned in the introduction, I am a consultant for Molecule, which has provided a grant for this book. Molecule makes excellent mattresses that I and my family members use. Other fans include Mike Phelps (a swimmer who won twenty-eight Olympic medals during his career) and his wife, Nicole, who are quoted in an ad saying they sleep better because their Molecule mattress regulates their body heat and core temperature.

It is important to stress that the specific brand of mattress a person chooses is a personal matter. There is no such thing as a "perfect" mattress for everyone. Fortunately, there are many excellent options, and most have money-back guarantees. Since a mattress is a piece of furniture you will be spending a third of your life on, I advise doing your own research and trying them out yourself. For guidance, many product reviews are available online. My comments are not meant to be a product review but, simply, a guide for what to look for and focus on.

Maxillomandibular advancement (MMA) surgery for sleep apnea. MMA surgery is an extensive procedure done by an oral and maxillofacial (OMF) surgeon to help treat obstructive sleep apnea (OSA). In performing the procedure, the OMF surgeon will break the jaw in four places—two spots on either side of the upper jaw, two on either side of the lower jaw—and then pull everything forward a few millimeters. The surgeon will then insert metal plates, which keeps everything in place as the bones grow together. This procedure increases the amount of space in the mouth by taking the tongue away from the back of the throat and making a larger area for the air to flow through. It can be curative for OSA, but I will usually not recommend the surgery unless the OSA is quite severe and there are no other options.

Meditation practices are known to have a positive impact on psychological well-being and sleep, and they are something I always discuss with my patients. Fortunately, there are many resources to turn to for instructions, including apps (Headspace and Calm, to name two) and YouTube, where you can simply search for "mindfulness meditation" or "how to meditate."

Let's go through the basics. In a quiet environment with the lights off, sit at the edge of the bed or in a chair. You can have soft music playing if you like, or do it in silence. Close your eyes, place your hands on your lap, and keep your eyes closed.

Start by breathing in through your nose and out through your mouth, nice and slow, and focus on your breathing. You can imagine images of air moving into your nose and out through your mouth, if that helps. Alternatively, you can say in your mind "in" as you breathe in and "out" as you breathe out.

As you're focusing on the breathing, you're probably going to have thoughts about other things. The important piece to remember is *not* to try to block out these extraneous thoughts, but rather, just acknowledge them, and then gently refocus on your breathing. Eventually, as you relax your mind, you will begin to feel the muscles in your body start to relax as well.

Start with the eyes and forehead muscles, next focus on your neck and shoulders, and then work your way down progressively, slowly relaxing each muscle as you continue to concentrate on breathing. If you try meditation for one minute daily, and then maybe work up to ten or fifteen minutes, you will see a benefit. It takes time to "perfect," so try to not be discouraged if your mind wanders.

I recommend that you make mindfulness meditation part of your bedtime ritual instead of watching TV or working on your computer. It can also be used in the middle of the night to help you get back to sleep.

Melatonin. A hormone produced by the pineal gland in the brain, melatonin synchronizes the sleep–wake cycle with night and day. Darkness prompts the pineal gland to start producing and secreting melatonin into the bloodstream, while light, especially sunlight and blue light (see "Sunlight" and "Blue light"), causes it to stop.

Melatonin is available as an over-the-counter supplement, and it can be very effective for insomnia. I may recommend an immediate-release version of melatonin—perhaps 1–3 mg taken thirty minutes before bedtime if someone has trouble falling asleep and a time-release version (same dose) if a patient has trouble staying asleep. There has been some recent controversy with melatonin insofar that the American Academy of Sleep Medicine is cautioning doctors from recommending it to patients willy-nilly. While I totally believe in melatonin, I agree that the purity of various supplements may be suspect, so you need to get it from a trustworthy source. In children, melatonin may possibly affect hormones. One thing is for sure: melatonin should not be used as a cure-all. If there is persistent trouble with sleep, seeing a sleep specialist and possibly undergoing a sleep test would be absolutely needed. As with any supplement, you need to talk with your doctor before starting it.

Memory and sleep are closely intertwined—both short-term memory and long-term. Not getting enough quality and quantity of sleep harms cognitive performance and results in reductions in memory, attention, and processing speed. In college and medical school, there were many times I would be up all night studying. However, in the early morning, I found that I was not able to remember much of what I studied. It would not be until I took a short nap that I could remember anything. (I *do not* recommend this, by the way, but it is a powerful, albeit unpleasant way of demonstrating how sleep is needed for memory.) Sleep helps us to consolidate and store important information we have taken in each day, and it helps us discard information we do not need. Based on what we know about the glymphatic system (see "Glymphatic system"), if we are not getting enough deep sleep, toxic proteins can build up in our brain—a situation which may predispose or contribute to dementia down the road.

Menopause. The two major hormones in women, estrogen and progesterone, play a role in sleep apnea and insomnia. When a woman begins to go through menopause (the "perimenopausal" period), these hormones begin to decline, and the result can be night sweats and hot flashes (see "Hot flashes and night sweats/hormone therapy"), which may disrupt sleep. Once menopause begins, the risk of sleep apnea also increases.

Premenopausal women are protected against sleep apnea; once estrogen and progesterone are no longer present, the risk to women almost reaches the level of men. When estrogen is gone, fat tissue may become deposited in the neck area (microscopically, not that someone could see it). With more fat tissue in the neck area, the airway gets smaller, which can increase the risk of sleep apnea. Progesterone also has many effects on the body, including its role as a respiratory stimulant; without it, a post-menopausal woman may not breathe as deeply in sleep, which can increase the risk of sleep apnea, especially when combined with the lack of estrogen.

Hormone replacement therapy (HRT) may relieve many symptoms of menopause, but that relief comes at possible risk, including breast cancer, stroke, and dementia. That being the case, HRT is a topic worth discussing with your OB/GYN practitioner.

Middle-of-the-night insomnia. Typically, there are two major causes for middle-of-the-night insomnia: one physical and the other mental. The physical includes breathing stoppages during the night (sleep apnea), abnormal movements during the night (such as periodic limb movements, see "PLMS—periodic limb movements of sleep"), prostate issues in a man, hormone changes in a woman, or even pain. Mental problems include anxiety, stress, or depression. If any of these issues are present, we need to address them to improve sleep. People often do other things in the middle of the night that keep them awake, including looking at the clock and checking their smartphone. It's best to try to avoid these. I urge my patients to listen to soft music or a podcast, do light reading, or meditate until they feel sleepy and then try to get back to sleep (see "CBT-I—Cognitive behavioral therapy for insomnia").

One other reason is not being aligned with your body clock (see "Circadian rhythm"). What I mean is if your body clock tells you to be asleep from 11:00 p.m. to 7:00 a.m., and instead you fall asleep at 9:00 p.m., your sleep at night *will* become disrupted, and it's likely you will wake up early and be unable to fall back asleep. Consistent sleep and wake times are important.

Military method. During World War II, the US Navy Pre-Flight School created a routine to help pilots fall asleep quickly. It took about six weeks of practice for the pilots to master the procedure, but they did over time, and it apparently worked—even after many cups of coffee and the sound of gunfire in the background.

The military method consists of the following steps:

- Relax your entire face, including the muscles inside your mouth.
- Drop your shoulders to release the tension, and let your hands drop to the side of your body.
- Exhale, relaxing your chest.
- Relax your legs, thighs, and calves.
- Clear your mind for ten seconds by imagining a relaxing scene.
- If this doesn't work, try saying the words "don't think" over and over for ten seconds.

Multiple sleep latency test (MSLT). This is a diagnostic test that measures how quickly a person falls asleep. It consists of four or five twenty-minute nap opportunities set two hours apart, often following an overnight sleep test (polysomnogram, PSG). The level of sleepiness is based on the premise that people will fall asleep faster the sleepier they are. The MSLT is used to test for hypersomnia (excessive daytime sleepiness) and the conditions that cause it: narcolepsy and idiopathic hypersomnia. One other piece of information that MSLT tests provide is whether the patient will enter REM sleep, which typically takes about ninety minutes. If someone gets into REM sleep during a twenty-minute nap, it is typically abnormal; if this happens twice in the context of excessive sleepiness during an MSLT, it is diagnostic of narcolepsy.

N

Naps. In nature, people normally have a dip in energy levels around lunchtime, which is why many countries have siestas; taking a short nap in the early afternoon can help with sleep deprivation from the night before. The problem is that some people sometimes nap too late or too long. For example, let's say after dinner, a person is watching the news on the couch and they fall asleep for fifteen minutes. Seems like an innocuous thing, right? But that short nap can prevent a person from being able to fall asleep at nighttime. Normally, sleep pressure (see "Sleep pressure") builds up over the course of a day, and that helps us fall asleep at night. A nap may reduce that sleep pressure. What I usually recommend patients do if they are going to nap is to do it early in the day. I also recommend a nap of fifteen to thirty minutes. When you nap longer than that, there is a good chance you are going to go into a deep sleep (see "Delta wave sleep"), which can leave you feeling worse after (see "Sleep inertia").

To summarize, naps can a natural, nice way of giving yourself a boost of energy, but they should be as early as possible, as well as short and sweet.

Narcolepsy is a chronic condition that is sometimes portrayed on TV and in movies as a comedic situation in which somebody falls asleep while driving or in a meeting, class, and so on. It certainly can present that way, but it's usually a little subtler.

People who have narcolepsy are tired in the daytime and have poor sleep at night. It's often combined with hallucinations when they are falling asleep or waking up, where they may see things moving across the room or shadows coming at them. Or they may have sleep paralysis, where they wake up in the middle of the night and are unable to move, as well as possibly having these hallucinations simultaneously.

They may also have another symptom called cataplexy, which is a loss of muscle strength in the context of an emotional trigger. If somebody gets very angry or is laughing hard about something, they may find that their knees buckle or their head falls forward and they can't lift it up. On other occasions, they may not be able to hold a cup in their hand. Or, in severe cases, they may drop to the ground. It could look very distressing to outside observers, who may think the person is having a seizure or is fainting. The person does not lose consciousness but loses muscle strength. After about a minute or two, the muscle strength returns and they are back to normal.

In cases where we suspect patients have narcolepsy, we often have them do a special overnight sleep test, followed by a nap test the next day (see "Polysomnography" and "Multiple sleep latency test [MSLT]").

Narcolepsy comes from either genetic predisposition (a family member may have similar symptoms), from a viral illness as a child, or for reasons that we do not know yet. There are two types: type 1 has the sleepiness, disrupted sleep, hallucinations, sleep paralysis, *and* cataplexy that we talked about earlier, and type 2 has all the symptoms but *without* cataplexy. In patients with narcolepsy type 1, there is a loss of a hormone called orexin (or hypocretin), which helps to stabilize sleep and wakefulness. When it is missing, sleep and wake tend to intrude onto one another, and cataplexy is a form of this intrusion. With type 2, we are not sure what exactly is causing the symptoms.

In either case, we treat narcolepsy in several ways. We often start by giving patients a wake-promoting agent or a stimulant medication to wake them up in the daytime (see "Wake promoting agents" and "Stimulant medications"); this usually helps to some degree, but they still may have disrupted sleep. The next step typically is to add gamma hydroxybutyrate (see "Gamma hydroxybutyrate") in the form of Xyrem or Xywav. The combination of a medication in the daytime to help with wakefulness and a medication at night to help the patient sleep more deeply usually does the trick. Sometimes, we have to mix and match medications and/or treat other problems like anxiety and depression, which often go along with narcolepsy.

Nasal EPAP. When *Let's Talk About Sleep* was published in 2018, a new technology called Provent had been introduced for the treatment of snoring and OSA. Ultimately (and unfortunately), it failed.

Provent, which used microvalve technology to keep the airway open, consisted of two adhesive patches that were worn over the nostrils during sleep. These patches would allow the patient to breathe in freely; but when breathing out, the valve would close and the breathed-in air would be directed toward the back of the throat, opening the airway until the start of the next breath. This is called EPAP, which stands for expiratory positive airway pressure—in simple English this means the patient is basically acting as their own CPAP. Each breath provides the pressure to keep the airway open.

Bongo Rx, ULTepap, and Optipillows are newer, better "versions" of Provent. While not covered by commercial insurers or Medicaid/Medicare, they are available for veterans via the VA system. Some data suggest that they work, but more robust and longer trials are needed.

Natural substances. There are many natural substances—either food itself or supplements—that can help promote sleep. Here is a list of some of the more popular ones:

- Kiwi contains a high concentration of serotonin, a precursor for the hormone melatonin that regulates your sleep–wake cycle.
- Pumpkin seeds. One ounce of pumpkin seeds contains 37 percent of your daily needs for magnesium, a mineral linked with healthy sleep.
- Cheese. If a warm glass of milk doesn't sound appealing, grab a few cubes of cheese, a protein-packed snack that is full of calcium, magnesium, and tryptophan—all of which may aid in a good night's sleep.
- Tart cherry juice. Tart cherries have a high dietary melatonin concentration, and they have also been shown to exhibit anti-inflammatory characteristics that may be beneficial in improving sleep quality.
- Rice. A study of Japanese men and women found that a high rice consumption was significantly associated with good sleep. Brown rice, which is high in fiber, is one way to go.

- Nuts. Almonds, walnuts, and pistachios contain melatonin, along with magnesium and zinc, which all together can help you get a better night sleep.
- Lavender oil is derived from the flowers of *Lavandula angustifolia* and is the most frequently recommended essential oil to aid sleep. It can be directly inhaled, used in bath products, applied to the skin as a massage oil, or taken by mouth as a capsule.
- Lemon balm, a member of the mint family, was used as far back as the Middle Ages to reduce stress and anxiety, promote sleep, improve appetite, and ease pain and discomfort from indigestion.
- L-theanine is an amino acid found in green tea, black tea, and certain types of mushrooms. When taken at night, it may help people relax, get to sleep more easily, and sleep more deeply.
- L-tryptophan, an amino acid found in red meat, poultry, eggs, dairy, nuts, seeds, and bananas is crucial in the production of serotonin, a chemical in the brain that affects mood and may help with conditions like anxiety and sleep disorders.
- Magnesium is believed to aid sleep by calming down the central nervous system. Good sources of magnesium include leafy green vegetables, nuts, seeds, legumes, and whole grains. Many people take magnesium supplements before bed.

Other substances thought to improve sleep include passion-flower, SAMe (S-adenosyl-L-methionine), tulsi tea, valerian, and chamomile tea. Like anything you read in this book, it is paramount that you have a consultation with your medical provider to ensure that these substances are safe for you.

Nicotine, a naturally produced substance of tobacco plants, is widely used recreationally. Since it is well-known that smoking is bad for us, I will not belabor the point, but it is important to review how it affects our sleep. Nicotine, whether it be from vaping, cigarettes, cigars, or gum, is a stimulant and part of the "Big Three," as I call them, of poor sleep (alcohol and caffeine being the others). While some swear by the relaxation that nicotine products provide, the fact is because of their stimulant nature, they will make it difficult to initiate sleep and will disrupt it. As I said, we should not smoke, vape, and so on, but if we absolutely need to use a nicotine product, it should be done so as early in the day as possible.

Nightmares are unpleasant dreams that can cause a strong emotional response in the mind—one that typically wakes us out of sleep. They are usually benign occurrences, but treatment may be needed when they happen regularly, as they can interfere with sleeping patterns and cause insomnia.

The word *nightmare* has its roots in the Old English *mare*, which is a mythological demon or goblin who torments others with frightening dreams. Because dreaming happens in REM sleep, that is where nightmares occur. And because periods of REM sleep become progressively longer as the night progresses, a nightmare will most often wake us out of sleep in the early-morning hours.

What triggers a nightmare? There are a lot of possibilities, including stress, anxiety, prior trauma (see "Trauma-associated sleep disorder [TSD]"), sleeping in an uncomfortable position, having a fever, and eating before going to sleep. It is of major importance to know that sleep apnea can trigger them as well. Dreams of being underwater, drowning, or not getting enough air are common, and since a patient is actually *not* getting enough air during sleep apnea, this seems to make sense.

Usually, reassurance is all that some needs to combat nightmares, but reducing stress levels, developing bedtime routines that are relaxing, and ensuring adequate rest are all potential treatments. Avoiding substances that can affect sleep (especially alcohol, nicotine, and caffeine), as well as keeping a consistent schedule, can also lower nightmare frequency. If they happen repeatedly, a referral to a sleep specialist may be needed, as may a sleep test (see "Polysomnography"), medications, or other psychological treatments.

The famous psychoanalysts Sigmund Freud and Carl Jung felt that nightmares are the brain's way of re-experiencing a stressful event from the past, and thus therapy could be helpful. When recurrent nightmares occur as a result of post-traumatic stress disorder (PTSD), a potential treatment called imagery rehearsal may be useful. Therapists will ask patients to come up with positive alternative outcomes to the nightmares and then to mentally rehearse those outcomes while awake; the patients are to remind themselves before bed what these outcomes should be. This technique may even improve daytime symptoms of PTSD.

In severe cases, we may use medications. Prazosin is probably the best, most known, and most widely used, but there are others (mostly in the psychiatric realm). And we cannot forget about sleep apnea. If it is present, it must be treated. Finally, some sleep aids may actually cause nightmares, and melatonin (of which I am a fan) can be in that category. Unfortunately, I have had to take a few patients off melatonin for this reason.

Night sweats can be caused by many different conditions and medications. They can come from hormonal changes (see "Hot flashes and night sweats/hormone therapy"), sleep apnea, infections, alcohol use, certain antidepressants, and clinical anxiety, to name a few. As I say throughout this book, it important to look into the underlying causes of problems like night sweats, and, in some cases, a sleep test may be of use.

Nocturia is the urge to urinate in the middle of the night. In many cases in men, it is related to prostate issues, but it is not always. In a good proportion, the real culprit is sleep apnea (OSA). The repetitive stoppages of breathing lead to mini awakenings, which then allow the signal from the bladder to get to the brain; this then leads the person to think "I need to empty my bladder." Normally they would sleep through it, but because of the sleep apnea at least partially waking them up, the person gets out of bed and urinates.

The other issue is that when someone has sleep apnea and is struggling to breathe through the night, pressure changes occur in the chest cavity, which result in the release of a hormone called atrial natriuretic peptide (ANP), a diuretic, which increases the need to urinate as well. Finally, it is important to note that water and liquid intake before bed can contribute to this. Usually, one to two hours or so before bed would be a good time to stop liquid intake (if nocturia is a problem), but it is still important to drink the recommended eight glasses of water per day.

NREM, or non-REM sleep, is the less glamorous sibling of REM (see "REM sleep"), but it is the main component of our sleep. We spend only 20–25 percent of our night in REM and the remainder in NREM (and yes, the naming is not very creative).

NREM sleep is broken into three stages. Stage 1, or N1, is very light sleep—the kind you would experience if you fell asleep in a meeting or on a subway; it is unrefreshing and very easy to wake up from. Non-REM stage 2, or N2, is the baseline of our sleep, the place our brain always returns throughout the night. Then there is non-REM stage 3, called delta wave sleep, which is very deep and hard to wake up from, which is why nature put it in the first half of the night (see "Delta wave sleep").

We have more REM sleep in the second half of the night and more delta wave sleep in the first half. If you've ever taken a long nap in the afternoon—say, two hours or so—you will probably wake up feeling worse than you did when you went to sleep. That's because your brain went into delta wave sleep, which is very difficult to wake up from (see "Sleep inertia").

The major differences between REM and delta wave sleep are important to recognize. REM sleep is essentially dream sleep; by spending time in dream sleep, we are able to form and store memories and improve our overall cognitive abilities. Delta wave sleep, on the other hand, seems to improve bodily functions: growth hormone is produced during this stage of sleep, and what happens during this period can have implications on muscle growth and organ repair.

This said, there is no such thing as "unimportant" sleep. The brain and the body need both REM and NREM (especially delta wave) sleep. The interplay between these two forms of sleep gives us sleep cycles, and this, in turn, forms the basis for the wonderful things that proper sleep does for us.

OSA—Obstructive sleep apnea. *Apnea* means not being able to breathe, so *sleep* apnea means not being able to breathe during sleep. Obstructive sleep apnea, or OSA, is the most common form of sleep apnea, which is thought to affect 20–30 percent of men and 10–15 percent of women in North America, though many cases are still undiagnosed. As society ages and gets heavier, OSA is almost certainly going to become even more prevalent.

When we are awake, the brain signals the upper airway to stay open; this includes the tongue, the tonsils, the uvula (the "punching bag" in the back of the throat), and the soft palate (the back part of the "roof" of the mouth). When we fall asleep, our muscles relax, which results in the airway becoming smaller.

When someone has unobstructed breathing in sleep, it means that the airway, even though it is a little smaller than when awake, is still wide open. In the case of snoring, the airway is tighter, either from weight (fat tissue on the neck), genetics, nasal congestion, smoking, alcohol, or other factors. As inhaled air rushes by when this person breathes in, it becomes very turbulent and causes the soft tissues to vibrate quickly, which results in the sounds of snoring. Snoring by itself is usually not harmful, but it could be a marker of OSA (but not everyone who snores has OSA, and not everyone who has OSA will snore).

When the airway closes off completely, we have an apnea caused by the obstruction. OSA, by definition, is tissue obstructing the airway for at least ten seconds. Contrary to popular belief, a person will not "choke to death" in this situation. Rather, the apnea triggers the brain to either wake up, go into lighter sleep, move the body, gasp for air, or otherwise do something to improve the blockage. This does not cause harm when it happens only once or twice, but after years and years of this happening nightly, problems may arise. Someone with OSA may be sleeping a full eight hours per night, but because his or her airway is repeatedly closing through the night, the quality of his or her sleep may be so impaired that they wake up totally unrefreshed and there may be health consequences.

Many people with OSA complain of grinding their teeth (bruxism). They also may have morning headaches. Some complain of needing to wake up to urinate through the night (which in many cases is falsely blamed on prostate issues), and there can be gastric reflux symptoms like heartburn. Over the years, serious cases of OSA have effects on blood pressure, blood sugar, and bodyweight, and can lead to atrial fibrillation (a-fib), heart attacks, strokes, diabetes, and even cancer.

Even in those who are very thin, OSA can still be present. It is important to note that the anatomy/physiology of the upper airway in someone with OSA tends to be "tight," which can set them up for airway closures in sleep. In some OSA patients, this has little to do with weight, but is rather based on age and genetics.

Having OSA can make it difficult to lose weight. This has to do with two hormones the body makes, leptin and ghrelin: leptin is made by our fat cells and tells us it is time to stop eating, whereas ghrelin is made by our stomach and tells us we are hungry. When sleep is disrupted because of OSA, these hormones get out of whack and can make it harder to control our appetite. Once OSA is treated, it may realign these hormones, which may raise energy levels and lead to an increased desire/ability to exercise. Both of these would potentially bring about weight loss.

Like insomnia, OSA gets more frequent as we get older—in both in men and women. Premenopausal women are protected against OSA, thanks to two other hormones: estrogen and progesterone. Once their production is stopped during menopause, the risk of having OSA in women almost reaches the level of men (see the entries for "Estrogen" and "Progesterone").

We characterize OSA by how often the airway closes each hour over the course of a night's sleep; this is determined by either an in-lab test (see "Polysomnography") or a home test (see "Home sleep testing"). Fewer than five events per hour is normal. If you took a thousand people at random and had them do a sleep test, the majority would have two or three events per hour, and believe it or not, this is not a big deal. Mild OSA consists of five to fifteen stoppages of breathing per hour; moderate OSA is fifteen to thirty stoppages per hour; and severe OSA is more than thirty stoppages per hour.

People who have mild and perhaps moderate OSA for a period of time are not usually affected in a major way health-wise, but people suffering with the moderate–severe and the severe form are at risk for other health concerns as we said above. After ten or fifteen years, OSA can have a big impact on mortality. We're talking about cardiovascular illness, strokes, heart attacks, and so on. It's a serious condition because it can take years off a person's life. The bottom line is if there is a possibility you have OSA, get tested.

Parasomnias refer to all forms of abnormal movements and sensations that occur near or during sleep. They include nightmares, sleepwalking, REM sleep behavior disorder, sexsomnia, exploding head syndrome, and hypnagogic and hypnopompic hallucinations—all of which are discussed in individual sections in this book. We break them down into those that occur during REM sleep (REM behavior disorder, sleep paralysis, and nightmares) and ones occurring in NREM sleep (sleep talking, sleepwalking, sleep terrors, and the like).

Performance anxiety. Let's say you are about to give a talk, or you are about to perform on stage or play a game, and you get nervous. You are nervous that you are not going to be able to perform well, which, unfortunately, can make it true. When it comes to sleep, insomnia patients may develop performance anxiety, which can make it very difficult to fall asleep; this then fuels the anxiety further for subsequent nights, and so on. This results in a vicious cycle where it's almost impossible to sleep.

We deal with this through behavioral modification and medications. These are mentioned throughout this book, but treatments such as cognitive behavioral therapy for insomnia (see "CBT-I—Cognitive behavioral therapy for insomnia") are useful, as is the use of hypnotics (see Hypnotics [sleep aids]) when needed. Another technique we sometimes use is called paradoxical intention. To try to reduce the performance anxiety, we tell people to say to themselves, "I want to stay awake, I want to stay awake, I want to stay awake" instead of "I want to get to sleep" or "I need to sleep." As the name suggests, paradoxically, this can reduce the anxiety and help induce sleep.

Pillows. Like mattresses and bedding (see "Mattresses" and "Bedding/ sheets"), the right pillow can play a major role in getting healthy sleep. Instead of a product review which you can easily find online from reputable sources, I will take this opportunity to review the basic principles you should use when choosing a pillow. It is, of course, very subjective, and you might be best served trying them out before deciding on one particular brand. Fortunately, many manufacturers offer a trial period that enables you to send it back if you don't like it.

A bed pillow can cost anywhere from ten dollars to hundreds or even thousands of dollars for some of the luxury ones, but among the highest rated pillows in a *U.S. News & World Report*, the average price was about sixty-seven dollars. Remember, like all things, higher price doesn't necessarily mean it is the right one for you.

The position you sleep in is a very important factor to consider when shopping for a new pillow. For example, side sleepers typically need thicker pillows to maintain the neutral position of their neck while lying on their side, while back sleepers require a less thick pillow (a thicker pillow will push the neck into a more flexed position). Those who sleep on their stomach should look for a thin pillow that provides enough support to prevent the head from tilting downward (but not so much that the head is forced up and back). For those of you who switch around during the night, an adjustable pillow might well be the answer.

I usually tell my patients to try to sleep in the fetal position, on the side, with the hips and knees at a ninety-degree angle. This is the most neutral position, and if someone is troubled by snoring or sleep apnea, it may reduce those problems—certainly compared to sleeping on the back. Sleeping on your stomach is okay for sleep apnea, but it may result in a stiff neck or back. For side sleepers, I usually recommend the firmer/ thicker pillow as mentioned above. I also feel that a pillow between the legs would be useful, as well as one of those long body pillows to hug.

If you suffer from chronic neck pain, using the right pillow can provide some relief. If you're lying on your side and your pillow is too high or too low, your neck will be kinked to one side or another for the duration of the night, which may lead to neck pain throughout the next day. The ideal pillow is one that is supportive enough to align your spine and soft enough to relieve pressure.

As for materials, there is also no right option for everyone, but here are a few things to consider: if you tend to sleep hot, you might want to avoid pillows that are made of a solid piece of memory foam, as foam tends to retain heat; instead, choose one that allows for more airflow. Avoiding down might be preferable for some people, due to the possibility of allergies, feathers poking out from the pillow, or wanting to avoid animal products.

Overall, you should replace your pillow when it's no longer supporting your head and neck properly. Down or down-alternative pillows should be replaced every one to two years, but pillows made of latex or bamboo can last a bit longer. A good rule of thumb is comfort: if you're constantly waking up with a crick in your neck, a headache, or allergy symptoms, it's probably time for a new pillow.

PLMS—periodic limb movements of sleep is a condition that involves repetitive and involuntary movements usually of the legs (but sometimes of the arms) during sleep. Symptoms range from a small amount of movement in the ankles and toes to the frank kicking of legs, which may or may not be noticed by a bed partner, who may often say that they see "leg twitching" during the night. The patients themselves are often not aware that they suffer from PLMS, but it would be apparent during an overnight in-lab sleep test (see "Polysomnography").

If the limb movements cause sleep disruption or result in unrefreshing sleep or daytime sleepiness, we refer to the condition as periodic limb movement disorder (PLMD). More than 80 percent of people with RLS also experience PLMS (see "Restless legs syndrome [RLS]"), and it is more common in older people, especially women. Like RLS, we see PLMS in conditions such as narcolepsy, sleep apnea, those with lower back or nerve problems (like sciatica), heart disease, and in men and women who do shift work. The use of caffeine, alcohol, or nicotine can make it worse, as can stress. The way to treat PLMS or PLMD is similar to the way we treat RLS (checking iron and ferritin and replacing it if needed; additionally, the use of medications if needed).

Polysomnography. A polysomnogram (PSG) is a comprehensive test used to diagnose sleep disorders. Often referred to as a sleep study, polysomnography records your brain waves, the oxygen level in your blood, and your heart and breathing rate, as well as your eye and leg movements during the night.

The test may be done in a sleep unit within a hospital or at a sleep center. Sometimes you may be able to do the study at home. Home testing uses a limited number of sensors to focus primarily on diagnosing obstructive sleep apnea (OSA). While it's typically performed at night, polysomnography can be done during the day to accommodate shift workers.

One aspect of PSG testing that often comes up are the questions patients ask, such as "What if I can't sleep?" or "What if the sleep apnea (or whatever condition we are looking for) doesn't happen that night?" While these are totally legitimate concerns, my response is typically along the lines of (1) if it exists, we usually will see it; (2) don't worry about having a "perfect" night, as we tend to get enough information in most cases; and (3) if we need to, we can have you take a supplement (like melatonin) or a medication to reduce some of the pre-test anxiety.

These days, many commercial insurance companies will not approve a PSG outright. Therefore, we tend to do a home sleep test first. If it is completely normal, we are then "allowed" to perform the PSG. If we are looking for garden-variety OSA, a home test is usually adequate.

Positional treatment for sleep apnea. People with sleep apnea often have breathing blockages when lying on their back, a condition known as positional sleep apnea. In these cases, breathing stops because gravity pulls the soft tissues and tongue down toward the back of the throat, which closes the airway as they sleep. Many times, the bed partners of my patients with positional sleep apnea will say something like, "I elbow him, he rolls over, and then he's fine."

Sometimes, however, an elbow in the ribs doesn't do the job. In these cases, more reliable treatment is needed, such as CPAP or a dental device (see the entries for "Continuous positive airway pressure [CPAP]" and "Mandibular advancement device [MAD]"). But when someone does not want to use these, we may turn to what is called a positional device. These are typically Velcro belts that have a hump in the back that prevents the person from rolling onto his or her back when worn during sleep. There are even electronic positional devices that vibrate, nudging the person off their back if they roll onto it. In the old days, people would get the same result by sewing tennis balls into T-shirts. Regardless of the method, there is a training aspect to making oneself sleep on the side or stomach. These devices may only be needed for a time, until the patient has trained themselves to avoid sleeping on their back.

If a person must lie on their back or it is the only comfortable position for them, being on an incline can help reduce snoring, sleep apnea, or even acid reflux (gastroesophageal reflux disease or GERD). A reliable method to create an incline would be to put bricks under the head of the bed, use a wedge pillow or, if it is an adjustable mattress, to raise the head up.

Post-prandial fatigue. Many people have an after-lunch feeling of tiredness, which is called post-prandial somnolence or fatigue. Our circadian signal—our internal clock—normally has a dip in the early afternoon, which is why we get more tired then. It's also why people in many other countries have siestas built into their daily routines. With the typical American diet (excess carbs, not enough vegetables), this signal can be magnified. And, of course, if there is a condition of hypersomnia (e.g., OSA or narcolepsy), this signal will also be magnified, which can lead to needing a nap after lunch or even more frequently.

Post-traumatic stress disorder (PTSD) is a mental disorder that develops following exposure to a traumatic event, such as warfare, sexual assault, or domestic violence. The symptoms may include disturbing thoughts or feelings, nightmares related to the events, insomnia, and increased fight or flight response. The sleep-related symptoms can be extremely distressing, including the acting out of dreams (see "REM behavior disorder [RBD]"). Treatment is designed to reduce the symptoms through the use of medication and therapy.

Recently, a new disorder called trauma-associated sleep disorder (TSD) has been described. It is associated with PTSD and results in an acting out of dreams, which makes it appear very similar to RBD. It is thought to be caused by hyperarousal, which is an increased fight or flight response to something that is a minimal threat—for example, a noise. This hyperarousal distinguishes TSD from RBD, in which we are more concerned about an impending neurologic illness. I am hopeful that with more research, we will have a better understanding of these disorders.

Predisposing, precipitating, and perpetuating factors of chronic insomnia: the "3P" model. First described by the late Dr. Arthur Spielman, the "3P" model of chronic insomnia is a way of understanding where long-term insomnia comes from (see "Chronic insomnia").

The first *P*, which stands for "predisposing," would include factors like a family history of insomnia or a personal history of anxiety or panic. The second *P*, for "precipitating," means something precipitates or triggers a bout of poor sleep—something, for example, like a divorce, a death in the family, or a job change.

At this point, the predisposition that was lying dormant becomes active, and yet sleep would have gone back to normal after this event concluded, if it were not for the third P. The third *P* stands for "perpetuating" factors—things like bad sleep habits, spending too much time in bed, and seeing bed as a place of stress rather than a place of sleep. That last P is where sleep hygiene comes into play (see "Sleep hygiene"). It is the area we focus on to improve sleep habits, in addition to other behavioral treatment (see "CBT-I—Cognitive behavioral therapy for insomnia") and medication if needed.

Pregnancy. As much as sleep is needed during pregnancy, it doesn't always come easily. During early pregnancy, daytime sleepiness and fatigue are common, but some specific sleep-related issues may emerge as well. Problems such as nausea and vomiting (morning sickness), frequent urination, physical discomfort (such as tender breasts and back pain), and fetal movements all can disrupt a pregnant woman's sleep. Actual sleep disorders such as sleep apnea and restless legs syndrome (see "Restless legs syndrome [RLS]") can be present as well.

During pregnancy, there is a two- to three-times higher chance that women will experience RLS—the risk is highest in the seventh to eighth months—but in 70 percent of women, it will improve or stop shortly after delivery. The reasons for RLS in pregnancy are not fully understood, but it is thought to be due to changes in iron and folate, genetic susceptibility, high estrogen levels, and the stretching or compression of nerves. Ideally, treatment of RLS in pregnancy does not include medications, but conservative measures such as iron supplements (if low), exercise, and stretching. The knowledge that the symptoms should improve once the child is born can also be a relieving factor.

An estimated 20 percent of pregnant women experience sleep apnea. It makes sense that sleep apnea would become more prominent during pregnancy, due to the normal body changes and weight gain that accompany it. But the condition often goes undiagnosed or undertreated because the symptoms overlap with common pregnancy side effects, such as headaches, heartburn, and morning nausea, as well as emotional changes such as anxiety and depression. Unfortunately, sleep apnea during pregnancy can lead to long-term health complications, including increased risk of high blood pressure, preeclampsia, gestational diabetes, or premature delivery. Untreated sleep apnea also increases the risk of requiring a C-section delivery, having complications with anesthesia, and enduring a longer labor. As with RLS, it is important to know that this can happen and to discuss this with your doctor.

During pregnancy, it is preferable to avoid sleeping on your back, which can put the weight of your uterus on your spine and back muscles. If sleep apnea is present, sleeping on your back can make it worse. The use of carefully placed pillows can help you get comfortable; placing a pillow between your bent knees or under your belly is worth trying. Many of the other relaxation and good sleep habits that are mentioned in this book are of importance during pregnancy.

Progesterone. Like estrogen, progesterone has many effects on a woman's body. For our purposes, its role as a respiratory stimulant is important. During and after menopause, when the production of progesterone drops dramatically, a woman may not be breathing as deeply in sleep, which can increase the risk of sleep apnea (see "OSA—Obstructive sleep apnea" and "Menopause").

Progressive muscle relaxation, also known as deep muscle relaxation, is a two-step procedure that helps you unwind—first, by tensing various muscles throughout your body for a count of ten, and then, by relaxing the muscles and imagining the tension leaving your body as you exhale. Typically, the person will go from head to toe over a period of fifteen minutes or so. As luck would have it, there are many great (and free) resources to be found online for those interested in learning how to perform progressive muscle relaxation.

Pulmonary hypertension is a condition that describes a gradual increase in blood pressure in the arteries of the lungs, which results in a shortness of breath, fainting, tiredness, chest pain, swelling of the legs, a fast heartbeat, and difficulty with exercise. While the cause is often unknown, risk factors include a family history, prior blood clots in the lungs, HIV/AIDS, sickle cell disease, cocaine use, chronic obstructive pulmonary disease, sleep apnea, living at high altitudes, and problems with the mitral valve of the heart. Unfortunately, there is currently no cure for pulmonary hypertension, but supportive measures such as oxygen therapy, diuretics, and certain medications may be used. I bring it up here because pulmonary hypertension may play a role in breathing disorders in sleep.

Questionnaires, sleep related. These are self-reported forms that patients fill out that reveal important information about their sleep health. There are several available, including the ones described here, as well as the Pittsburgh Sleep Quality Index and the Fatigue Severity Scale. Most are available online. If you have concerns about your sleep health or someone else's, I urge you to check them out.

The questionnaire used most often is the Epworth Sleepiness Scale. It consists of eight scenarios, such as "sitting and reading" and "watching TV," and the patient is asked to determine the likelihood that they would fall asleep in the given scenarios. Somebody who is very sleepy (from narcolepsy or sleep apnea, for example) may score very high, but somebody who has insomnia may score very low. It is not perfect, but it does allow us to gauge the relative sleepiness that a patient experiences at a given point in time and how effectively a particular treatment may be working.

The STOP-BANG Questionnaire is a measure of the risk for obstructive sleep apnea (OSA) that a patient may have. The letters stand for snoring, tired (fatigued, or sleepy), observed (observed you stop breathing or choking/gasping episodes), pressure (high blood pressure), BMI (Body Mass Index more than 35 kg/m^2), age (more than fifty years), neck (circumference more than sixteen inches), and gender (males are at higher risk). If a person answers "yes" to three or more, their likelihood of having OSA is significant.

Rebound insomnia is defined as trouble either getting to sleep or staying asleep that is worsened after an abrupt discontinuation of sleeping pills—the "rebound" part of it may result in the insomnia being worse than ever. Some sleeping pills, especially benzodiazepines (benzos), can result in physical dependence, where the person may need more and more of the medication to get the same effect (see "Hypnotics [sleep aids]"). If there is abrupt discontinuation of high doses, a withdrawal may occur, leading to changes in blood pressure, heart rate, and—in severe cases—seizures.

Rebound insomnia is not as scary as withdrawal, but it can be very unpleasant. A drug with a short half-life—one that is out of your system quickly, like Sonata or Ambien—may lead to more intense rebound insomnia, but it may resolve more quickly, often fading within a few days to a week after the medication is stopped. Longer-acting medications like Klonopin may not have as pronounced an impact of rebound insomnia, but it may take longer for the drug to fully leave your system, resulting in residual morning hangover effects.

If you are regularly taking a prescription or an over-the-counter substance to help you sleep, and you develop rebound insomnia as soon as you stop it, it may be tempting to believe that you really *need* that substance to sleep. It would be better to wean down slowly—ideally, with a doctor's guidance. This is of utmost importance in the case of benzos. Sleep aides play a role when needed in a person's sleep health, but I am a cautious user. While certain medications like Trazodone are fine for nightly use (if okayed by your doctor), there are others I am opposed to using this way (e.g., Xanax). But the bottom line is that prescription medications, over-the-counter substances, and even combinations need to be used judiciously and with the understanding that other facets of sleep health, such as behavioral modification (see "CBT-I—Cognitive behavioral therapy for insomnia") and treatment of conditions like sleep apnea, must be done in addition to just taking a pill.

Relaxing breath technique. The 4-7-8 breathing technique, also known as "relaxing breath," consists of a series of exercises that many people find help them get to sleep. Based on the ancient Indian practice *pranayama*, it is often described as a natural tranquilizer for the nervous system. It involves breathing in for four seconds, holding the breath for seven seconds, and then exhaling for eight seconds—a pattern designed to reduce anxiety. Some proponents claim that the method helps people get to sleep in as little as one minute.

Although there is limited scientific research to support the 4-7-8 method, a great deal of anecdotal evidence suggests that this type of deep, rhythmic breathing is relaxing and may help ease people into sleep. It consists of the following steps:

- Place the tip of your tongue against the ridge of tissue behind your upper front teeth.
- Close your mouth and inhale quietly through your nose for four seconds.
- Exhale completely and loudly through your mouth.
- Inhale and hold your breath for seven seconds.
- Exhale completely and loudly through your mouth for eight seconds
- Repeat for as long as it takes to get to sleep.

REM behavior disorder (RBD) is a condition that is typically seen in older patients in which the muscle paralysis that normally occurs in REM sleep no longer occurs (see "REM sleep"). This results in people acting out the things they are dreaming about, for example, dreaming about a boxing match results in the patient punching their bed partner or the wall while completely asleep. Please note: "attacking" a bed partner does not mean that there is an underlying desire to hurt them. RBD was first reported in 1986 by Dr. Carlos Schenck, a renowned sleep clinician, psychiatrist, and researcher at the Minnesota Regional Sleep Disorders Center, and our knowledge since then has grown by leaps and bounds.

RBD is important because the patient could hurt themselves or their bed partners, but the *real* reason we care about it is that there is a linkage to disorders in the Parkinson's disease category (neurodegenerative illnesses is a term for them). The link to the neurodegenerative illnesses is a hot topic of research, both for me personally and for many prestigious sleep labs around the world. Unfortunately, there is nothing we can do to stop this, but we can treat the symptoms. High-dose melatonin or low-dose Klonopin—either separately or together—work well in quelling those dream enactments. Sometimes, RBD is caused by antidepressants like SSRIs and tricyclic medications. If a person is taken off these medications, the RBD may stop, but not always. Again, this is a condition that we are learning more about, and we don't have all the answers yet.

An important point to mention is that RBD-type symptoms may be present in those with severe sleep apnea. Due to the repetitive stoppages of breathing, the body responds as if it is in danger, with arms flailing and even screaming. It can look very similar to that of a true RBD; in fact, the term we use is called "pseudo-RBD." Another condition to mention here is trauma-associated sleep disorder (see "Trauma-associated sleep disorder [TSD]"), which shares many similarities with RBD but does not have the same link to the neurodegenerative spectrum. Finally, patients with narcolepsy may report RBD; in those cases, which are usually with younger patients, we do not think of them as having neurodegenerative risk.

The bottom line is if someone is suspected of having RBD, a sleep evaluation and an in-lab PSG are needed.

REM rebound. When REM sleep (see "REM sleep" later) is chronically deprived, the brain will do what it can to make up for it. If somebody chronically smokes marijuana, for example, that will inhibit REM sleep; when the person does not use marijuana for a night or two, the brain will say, "I need more REM sleep," and it will go into REM full force. This REM rebound will include a much higher percentage of the night spent in REM, and the dreams will be much more intense, vivid, and often nightmarish. We see this not just with chronic marijuana users, but in any condition that reduces REM sleep—obstructive sleep apnea (see "OSA—Obstructive sleep apnea") being the most prominent. When an OSA patient is first placed on CPAP, they may also have REM rebound and then say things like, "I've never dreamed before, but now I do, and the dreams are very memorable." The point here is that we need REM sleep, and the brain will do what it can to make sure we don't go too long without it.

REM sleep, or rapid eye movement sleep, is essentially dream sleep; we believe it is responsible for memory storage, among other things. When the brain is in this special state, the body is normally prevented from acting out the dreams by being placed in paralysis. During this period of sleep, only three groups of muscles work—the diaphragm, which allows us to breathe; the eye muscles, which make the eyes dart back and forth rapidly (hence *rapid* eye movement sleep); and one of the muscles in the inner ear. Normally, we spend 20–25 percent of our night in REM sleep, spaced out in four or five periods across the seven to nine hours that the average person needs. REM sleep alternates with non-REM sleep (see "NREM, or non-REM sleep") during the night, and this back and forth is what we call sleep cycles (see "Sleep cycles").

REM sleep is very important for brain health and function, and there are several situations in which REM sleep is affected. Because the muscles are paralyzed during REM sleep, there is a much higher risk of obstructive sleep apnea (OSA). The airway goes from being relaxed in NREM sleep, to being totally flaccid in REM sleep, which may result in a much higher risk of airway closure. This is why many OSA patients tell us they never dream. Because the sleep apnea is so much worse in REM sleep, patients are never able to remain in it. However, once we start them on CPAP, REM sleep comes back full force (see "REM rebound").

An important situation to note is when the paralysis of REM sleep does not occur. In these cases, the body is basically allowed to act out the dreams of the brain. We call this "REM behavior disorder" (see "REM behavior disorder [RBD]"), and it is something that needs to be addressed.

REM sleep is very important for our brains and our sleep health, and its presence or absence can help us to determine if there are sleep-related problems that may have been hiding in plain sight.

Remede. In cases where someone has central sleep apnea (see "Central sleep apnea [CSA]"), there is a failure of the signal to breathe. The diaphragm, the main muscle that sits above our stomach, causes our lung cavity to expand and take a breath in when it is activated. There are situations in which the signal to activate becomes faulty and breathing will stop. This is not due to a blockage in the airway as seen with *obstructive* sleep apnea; rather, it's due to the diaphragm not being told to take a breath, which is called *central* sleep apnea (as in the central nervous system). This can be caused by several conditions, including heart failure. There are different ways we can deal with it: the first, being to treat the cardiac condition; after that, turning to therapies that use pressurized air (see "Continuous positive airway pressure [CPAP]" and "BPAP").

Recently, a newer therapy has emerged: "transvenous phrenic nerve stimulation," which goes by the brand name Remede and has been approved by the US Food and Drug Administration. Remede works by providing an electrical pulse to the nerve that controls the diaphragm (the phrenic nerve) during sleep, which causes you to take a breath. Used for moderate to severe central sleep apnea, the system produces a steady breathing pattern. Similar to the Inspire device (and other hypoglossal nerve stimulators), Remede involves a battery-powered pulse generator that is implanted under the skin in the upper chest.

Restless legs syndrome (RLS) is a condition in which uncomfortable sensations in the legs (and sometimes the arms) result in difficulty falling asleep. The four main symptoms, summarized by the acronym "URGE," consist of U for the urge to move, R for a feeling of restlessness, G for go (when the sufferer gets up and goes, the symptoms resolve), and E for evening (which is when the symptoms become problematic).

RLS is fairly common, affecting as much as 10–15 percent of the population. Symptoms can be anywhere from mild to incredibly severe, to the point where they can result in nights of lack of sleep. In about two-thirds of sufferers, these symptoms gradually worsen over time.

RLS can become part of a vicious cycle. If you don't sleep well or don't sleep enough, RLS becomes worse night after night. In many cases, we look for other issues that may occur in sleep—namely, sleep apnea or leg kicking during the night. We call these leg kicks "PLMS," or periodic limb movements of sleep (see "PLMS—periodic limb movements of sleep"). Both sleep apnea and PLMS can disrupt sleep, leading to a more "irritable" nervous system and thus making RLS even worse and more difficult to treat. I find when I see patients for a second or third opinion, usually the sleep apnea is the missing piece that has not been fully addressed. Treating the sleep apnea may make the treatment for RLS be more effective.

What is also not mentioned enough is that patients with RLS have higher rates of depression and anxiety disorders, which, when untreated, make the RLS harder to treat. And there is a strong link between RLS and attention deficit hyperactivity disorder (ADHD). RLS can occur in children and may be attributed to "growing pains." Children may have a difficult time describing the symptoms, but it is often apparent during an overnight sleep test.

In many cases, the cause of RLS is unknown, but there may be a genetic component. I often hear a patient say, "My mom had something like this." Additionally, pregnancy is big cause—particularly in the last trimester—and RLS often improves within four weeks after delivery (see "Pregnancy").

We can treat RLS in a couple of ways. We start with the conservative treatment, which consists of avoiding the "Big Three" (alcohol, nicotine, and caffeine) and certain medications that can cause the condition. I've had a few patients who were taking diphenhydremine (Benadryl or other similar, over-the-counter antihistamines) for allergies, itching, or insomnia, and who did not realize that these substances can make RLS worse. Stopping the substances helped.

Stretching before bed can be helpful. One particularly good stretch is a calf stretch up against a wall that is held for thirty seconds. This is followed by a few seconds of rest and then another repetition of stretching for thirty seconds, and so on. Doing the stretch five times or so before bedtime can be useful.

Doing engaging activities before bed can also be helpful. Some have suggested that video games, word puzzles, or talking (or even arguing) with a bed partner can help. While these are not great suggestions for insomnia, for RLS, they help to take a patient's mind off the symptoms.

Finally, some may benefit from physical therapy and/or things like taking hot or cold baths, whirlpool baths, applying hot or cold packs to the legs, massage, or vibratory or electrical stimulation of the feet and toes before bedtime. Similarly, regular exercise and relaxation techniques can also help.

We also look at the patient's iron levels, particularly in young menstruating women. They may have low iron levels, which itself can bring on RLS. The level that we are most concerned with is called ferritin, which is a blood marker of iron stores in the body. Usually, we want this level to be above 50 or 75 in an RLS patient (normal range in women is 11 to 307 micrograms per liter). (See "Ferritin.")

The use of daily medication is usually reserved for patients suffering symptoms at least three nights a week, but there are times when we will use medications on an as-needed basis. There are a few classes of drugs we use, and some of them are also used in insomnia or other conditions. Here is a list of the common ones:

- Dopamine-based medications are primarily used to treat Parkinson's disease (PD), although RLS has nothing to do with PD. They include two pills, ropinirole (Requip) and prami-pexole (Mirapex), as well as the patch rotigotine (Neupro). They are usually tolerated well, though the side effects can include nausea and dizziness. The problem with dopamine-based medications is more long-term. They can cause what is known as augmentation, which is apparent progressive worsening of RLS symptoms. This includes getting symptoms earlier in the day until, finally, the symptoms are present around the clock and/or occur in the arms or even the torso. Removing the person from all dopamine-related medications can solve the problem, although it can be uncomfortable in and of itself. Typically, we will add another medication as we are weaning or cutting off the dopamine. These medications can lead to compulsive behaviors like shopping or gambling, and stopping them can reverse these behaviors.
- Gabapentin-based medications. Gabapentin (Neurontin), while technically an antiseizure drug, is used by neurologists and other doctors for a variety of issues, including pain, headaches, and—you guessed it—RLS. In fact, it is usually my personal first choice, because the side effects are not terrible. The main thing

is that it can cause weight gain and may make sleep apnea a little worse in those who have it. Other side effects include dizziness and fatigue, as well as sleepiness (which is helpful in cases of sleep disturbance). Two cousins of gabapentin, called gabapentin enacarbil (Hortizant) and pregabalin (Lyrica), may also be useful; in some cases, they may be even more effective than gabapentin. I find that patients are often hesitant to try this out because of what they read online. This medication is extremely commonly prescribed, and despite what you may read, it is fairly safe (definitely safer than most others).

- Benzodiazepines are medications that also work on the GABA system and can treat many different conditions, including anxiety and muscle spasms. They can be very helpful when used safely in the right patient; side effects include daytime sleepiness and potential addiction (although this is low when it used as prescribed). The other potential issue is that they can also worsen sleep apnea.
- Opiates. In some severe cases, we might opt for opiate medications. These have gotten a bad reputation over the years (and rightfully so) but when used for a chronic condition like RLS (in very low doses), there is very little risk of addiction. We typically would start with methadone and see how the patient responds. As was true with the benzos, we need to make sure there is not untreated sleep apnea present. But for someone for whom nothing else works, this is a viable option.

Lastly, several underlying medical conditions—diabetes, nutritional deficiencies, kidney disease, thyroid disease, varicose veins, arthritis, back or knee problems, nerve damage (called neuropathy), or Parkinson's disease—can bring on or worsen RLS. As was the case with sleep apnea, these need to be addressed, or else the RLS will become much harder to manage. Dietary supplements to correct vitamin or mineral deficiencies may be recommended; one such example would be vitamin B12.

Like narcolepsy, RLS is sometimes portrayed as a comical condition. Also, like narcolepsy, it is not funny and can greatly impact a person's life. If any of the above hit home, talk with your doctor.

Revenge bedtime procrastination, a relatively new term, is something we have all done. Imagine getting pulled in a million directions after a long day: you sit down on your couch at 9:00 or 10:00 p.m., and even though you know you should be starting to wind down, you stay up, playing video games, binge watching a show, internet surfing, and so on—knowing that you will pay for it in the morning. This is called revenge bedtime procrastination. While the term has gained traction on social media, regular old bedtime procrastination has been around forever. The revenge part comes in if you're staying up out of frustration because work and other responsibilities have left you without any "me" time, which has occurred more so during the recent pandemic because the boundaries between work and home life have been distorted.

Many of the ways to combat revenge bedtime procrastination are discussed throughout this book, but here is a summary of four that I agree with:

- If you're working from home, create a "commute," even if it's simply taking a walk around the block. This will give you space and time to clear your head.
- Find new, upbeat nighttime activities. They could include turning off the TV and meditating for five to ten minutes, reading a book on paper, and listening to a podcast or soft music.
- Set an alarm that will tell you it's time for bed.
- Talk to a therapist or sleep specialist.

Second sleep. In the Middle Ages (medieval times), people reportedly slept in two phases (biphasic sleep), a process that led to what became known as "second sleep." This would entail going to sleep in the early evening, then waking up after four hours or so to do work, eat, and so on, and then going back to sleep for another few hours. With the coming of the Industrial Revolution came tighter work schedules, the emergence of artificial light, the use of caffeine, the introduction of clocks, and so on, so the two phases soon became one.

In more recent times, some have argued that the loss of these two sleep periods has done a disservice to our sleep and sleep health. However, there is little to no evidence that segmented sleep is better. If you are an inventor or an artist and are able to sleep whenever the mood grabs you, two-phase sleep may be fine (Edison and Da Vinci reportedly slept this way). But if you work a regular, nine-to-five job, trying this approach may leave you with a sleep schedule that gets farther and farther apart. You may not be able to get back to sleep for the second sleep, and as result, you would be tired at work. Or you may come home, take a nap, and then not be able to get to sleep at your normal bedtime, so you'd end up being sleep deprived at work. Thus, the cycle would continue. It is better to focus on the good sleep habits outlined in this book.

Selective serotonin reuptake inhibitors (SSRIs) are the most commonly prescribed form of antidepressants. They work by increasing the amount of serotonin in the brain, which eases the symptoms of anxiety and depression. They are relatively safe and typically cause fewer side effects than most other types of antidepressants. In treating anxiety and depression, SSRIs can reduce a major cause of insomnia. At the same time, one of their side effects causes difficulty with sleep. In other words, deciding whether to use SSRIs to deal with sleep is a balancing act— one you should discuss with your doctor or clinician.

Serotonin, a well-known molecule found throughout the brain, has a role in many brain functions such as memory, cognition, feelings of mood, sexual desire and function, appetite, sleep, memory and learning, temperature regulation, and social behavior. But a long-posed question in the scientific community has to do with serotonin's role in sleep: Does it promote sleep or promote wakefulness? A few years back, scientists at the California Institute of Technology found that serotonin is necessary for sleep in the zebrafish and mouse models. They theorized that the release of serotonin is a way for the brain to build up sleep pressure (see "Sleep pressure"); when the zebrafish and mice in the study lacked serotonin, they had reduced sleep pressure. While the studies were in animal models, it is believed that their production and release of serotonin are similar to that of our brains.

Setting your internal clock (circadian rhythm). Taking melatonin at bedtime and using sunlight or bright light in the morning can be a huge help in regulating one's internal clock. Same goes for keeping a strict bedtime and wake time, especially when going from weekdays to weekends.

Sexsomnia. A condition in which people engage in sexual activity while being asleep, it is similar to a sleepwalking episode but is confined to the bed. It is usually reported in men, but is probably under-reported overall, due to the possibility of embarrassment. Just like a sleepwalking episode, there is no recall of what happened. Typically, sexsomnia is a benign condition, but like all similar parasomnias (sleepwalking, sleep related eating disorder, etc.), we may want to search for an underlying sleep problem if it causes significant distress or occurs frequently.

Shift work disorder. Not everyone who works night shifts suffers from shift work disorder, but those who do often have difficulty sleeping when sleep is desired, and they find sleepiness when they desire to be wide awake. Additionally, they tend to have poor concentration, irritability, depression, and problems with interpersonal relationships. And most people who do shift work do not have access to healthy foods. They often rely on vending machines and the like, which is another potential cause for health problems.

Unfortunately, data suggest that performing shift work on a long-term basis also can lead to cancer and other potentially life-altering diseases. The reasons are varied, and while no one theory has been proven correct, it seems that a reduction in melatonin may play a role. When shift workers are exposed to light during the night shift, it prevents melatonin from being released into the brain, and we know that melatonin is a very strong antioxidant. When it is not produced, the body is essentially in a more inflamed state, and that can cause problems over long periods of time.

To help my patients combat the problems of shift work, I have them take melatonin (usually 1–3 mg) after the shift is over and when they are on their way home to get to sleep. If they are driving, I may have them wait until they actually get home before they take melatonin. It goes without saying that it is imperative for a shift worker to exercise extreme caution when on the road in a sleep-deprived state. As soon as they get out of work, night-shift workers should wear sunglasses and try to avoid the sunlight as much as possible. The reasons are (1) that sunlight is our strongest signal that it is time to be awake, and (2) being exposed to it shuts off melatonin.

When night-shift workers get home, they should have as dark an environment as possible, using blackout shades or eye masks. Getting quality sleep in the daytime can offset the bad effects of shift work, so daytime sleep becomes even more precious for these people. Sometimes, we will use prescription medications to promote sleep.

For work the next day, a good suggestion is to take a thirty-minute nap before the shift begins. Having scheduled naps during the shift would also be helpful, if possible, as would exposure to bright light before or in the early part of the shift. Caffeine can be very helpful at work, but sometimes we use prescription wake-promoting agents, such as modafinil (Provigil) or armodafinil (Nuvigil) to help keep these workers awake and alert at work. Finally, if the workers' shifts rotate, going forward would be ideal for him or her (later and later shifts) because going backward (earlier and earlier shifts) is a difficult adjustment for the body.

Sleep cycles, a term that is often misused, refers to the various stages our brain goes through when we fall asleep.

When asleep, the brain goes through cycles, or periods of non-rapid eye movement sleep (see "NREM, or non-REM sleep"), followed by a period of rapid eye movement sleep (see "REM sleep"); then there may be a brief awakening, or a move to lighter sleep. This process occurs in approximately ninety-minute blocks (which can range anywhere from 60 to 120 minutes), and each one of these blocks is a cycle. Typically, we have four or five of these cycles every night.

As the brain moves through NREM sleep in each cycle, it starts off with non-REM stage 1, or N1, which is very light sleep. The brain then moves into N2, which is the baseline of our sleep where we spend about 50 percent of our night. In N3, we see the deepest form of sleep, which we call delta wave or slow wave sleep. The brain moves through these three stages of NREM sleep and then ends with a period of REM.

As the night moves along, the time spent in N3 goes down and the time spent in REM goes up. REM takes about 25 percent of our night, and the time spent in it increases as each sleep cycle progresses. In a classic sense, we wake up out of REM sleep (otherwise known as dream sleep), which is why we remember our dreams.

Sleep cycles are part of what is called sleep architecture, a name that comes from how the sleep stages all look when seen together during a sleep test; if we add up the four or five sleep cycles that take place over the course of a night, it results in a certain, normal appearance that we would see on a graph (it almost looks like a skyline, hence "architecture"). When someone has a sleep disorder, the architecture may be affected, leading to poor quality sleep even if the quantity is fine.

Sleep diary. A sleep diary is an easy and useful way to track your sleep at home. It usually covers a two-week period and is most effective when you complete it on a daily basis. A sleep diary is a method you and your doctor can use to determine whether you are getting enough sleep and whether the quality sleep of sleep is sufficient. Insufficient or interrupted sleep can have serious health consequences, but the problems that impact sleep aren't always easy to identify. For that reason, a sleep diary is a valuable tool for monitoring sleep habits and documenting sleeping problems.

Although not all sleep diaries are identical, they commonly ask for information on the following details:

- bedtime and/or lights-out time
- wake-up time
- how long it takes to fall asleep
- the number and duration of sleep interruptions
- the number and duration of daytime naps
- perceived sleep quality
- consumption of alcohol, caffeine, and/or tobacco
- daily medications
- daily exercise

The sleep diaries I prefer can be found at the American Academy of Sleep Medicine's website: https://sleepeducation.org/resources/sleep -diary.

Sleep-disordered breathing (SDB). Also known as sleep-related breathing disorders, this is an umbrella term for a variety of problems with breathing during sleep, including obstructive sleep apnea (OSA), central sleep apnea (CSA), hypoventilation, and upper airway resistance syndrome (UARS), as well as other abnormalities of respiration during sleep, such as snoring and catathrenia. See the "Snoring" and "Catathrenia (nighttime groaning)" entries for more information.

Sleep efficiency refers to the percentage of time spent asleep while in bed. It is calculated by dividing the amount of time spent asleep (in minutes) by the total amount of time in bed (in minutes). A normal sleep efficiency is considered to be 85 percent or higher. Conditions in which the sleep is disrupted, such as sleep apnea, can make sleep efficiency worse. By contrast, idiopathic hypersomnia (see "Idiopathic hypersomnia [IH]") will typically show quite high sleep efficiency on an overnight polysomnogram sleep test.

Sleep hygiene refers to a collection of practices recommended for high-quality sleep. Improvement in this area is probably the best way to make an initial plan to combat insomnia. I know it sounds like I mean

"Keep your bedroom clean," but actually, sleep hygiene means keeping your bedtime habits "clean."

- The easiest place to start would be to shut off electronic devices that have a back-lit screen around thirty to sixty minutes before sleep time, and certainly not to use them in bed or if you wake up in the middle of the night.
- Use the bed and bedroom only for sleep and sex. If you feel the need to do anything else in bed, try reading a book or magazine on paper for up to fifteen to twenty minutes, or listening to soft music.
- Keep a strict sleep–wake schedule. This is important especially on the weekends, when many people sleep in. This can throw off your internal clock.
- Get regular exercise, ideally in the morning.
- Avoid caffeine after 1:00–2:00 p.m.
- Eliminate nicotine and reduce alcohol, especially close to bedtime (see "The "Big Three" of bad sleep").
- Getting sunlight in the morning can be useful to teach your brain that this is the time to be awake. I recommend twenty minutes or so (but not looking at the sun) to get your brain to shut off melatonin and wake itself up.
- Drink eight glasses of water throughout the day, but stopping a couple hours before bedtime would be important.
- Practice relaxation techniques (such as mindfulness meditation) regularly, both at bedtime and in the middle of the night as needed.
- Try to avoid napping. If you must nap, a siesta or a short thirty-minute nap as early in the day as possible is fine. One big no-no is an after-dinner snooze while watching TV, even if it's for only ten minutes or so; it can really screw up your brain's ability to get to sleep at the proper time later on.

Like many of the practices we talk about throughout this book, improving sleep hygiene will not transform your sleep overnight (pun intended). The important thing is to do your best and to be patient with it.

Sleep inertia is an abnormal condition that occurs upon awakening and refers to a strong desire to return to sleep; there may be also be impaired performance. The intensity and duration of sleep inertia vary based on a variety of situational factors, and some people can't shake that feeling for several hours. Typically, sleep inertia results because the brain has woken up out of N3 sleep (see "Delta wave sleep"), which normally occurs early in the night. If the brain is trying to make up for lost sleep during what is called a recovery night, sleep inertia may occur. During recovery nights, the brain essentially becomes more efficient and tries to get extra N3 sleep, which results in deep sleep occurring at the end of the night (which it normally would not), hence making it difficult to wake up. Similarly, if someone takes a nap in the daytime after not sleeping much the night before, the brain will attempt to get more N3 sleep and the nap will become very difficult to wake up from, especially if it is one to two hours long (or more). This is one reason we recommend naps be on the shorter side.

Sleep latency is a measure of how long it takes for the brain to move into a state of sleep. It would be increased in insomnia and decreased in conditions of hypersomnia (like narcolepsy). It can be measured during a multiple sleep latency test (see "Multiple sleep latency test [MSLT]") and helps us to determine the patient's level of sleepiness.

Sleep loss/deprivation. In the short term, the brain tries to make up for lost sleep by being more efficient during a recovery night or during a nap (see "Sleep inertia"). But this recovery mechanism only goes so far, and the consequences of sleep loss can be disastrous over long periods of time. For example, rats die after about two to three weeks of total sleep deprivation, which is similar to the life expectancy of rats undergoing total food deprivation (humans are more advanced than rats, of course, but you get the point). For us, chronic sleep deprivation leads to many changes, including elevations in inflammatory hormones, blood sugar, blood pressure, the likelihood of depression (and thus suicide risk), poor decision making (leading to car accidents and other preventable disasters), and overall reduced survival. Thus, it is important to get enough of both quality and quantity sleep.

Sleep paralysis is a condition that occurs when a person abruptly awakens from REM sleep (see "REM sleep"). Normally in REM sleep, our muscles are completely paralyzed, and if our mind partially wakes up but the body is still in REM sleep, there will be a frightening experience of being awake and paralyzed. There also may be dream imagery that feels real (again, from REM sleep, which is dream sleep).

Sleep paralysis can happen to anybody, and although it is scary, it is usually totally benign. But if it happens frequently (e.g., once per week), it could be a sign of sleep apnea or narcolepsy, and it probably should be evaluated further.

One point of interest here is that sleep paralysis has been put forth as a potential explanation for when people report they have been abducted by aliens. Think about it being paralyzed, half awake, with some dream imagery of being poked and prodded by an alien (see "Hypnagogic/hypnopompic hallucinations"), and it actually makes sense. This is not to say that I don't think aliens exist (I think they do), but that is a topic for another book.

Sleep positions. I often recommend my patients to try to sleep in the fetal position, on the side, with the hips and knees at a ninety-degree angle. This is a neutral position for the spine, assuming that the head is straight and not kinked to one side or another. If someone is troubled by snoring or sleep apnea, side sleeping may reduce those problems, especially when compared to sleeping on the back. To help this along, a pillow between the legs would be useful, as well as a long body pillow to hug (see "Positional treatment for sleep apnea").

Sleeping on your stomach is okay for sleep apnea, but it may result in a stiff neck or back. And sleeping on the back (supine) may be more comfortable for those with neck or lower back issues, but you have to think about whether snoring or sleep apnea is present. Being on your back allows gravity to pull the tongue to the back of the throat, which can worsen snoring and sleep apnea. If you must lie on your back and you have snoring, sleep apnea, or even acid reflux (see "Acid reflux"), sleeping on an incline or wedge pillow can help.

Sleep pressure is an unconscious biological response that makes us want to go to sleep. Without enough sleep pressure, it becomes difficult for us to initiate sleep or sleep for long. Basically, it is the idea that the longer the brain is awake, the stronger the drive is to get to sleep. That is why I do not recommend napping any time after the morning. Even if it is just a five-minute snooze on the couch after dinner, a nap can reduce the sleep pressure for the day, making it more difficult to get to sleep at night.

Sleep-related eating disorder, also known as sleep eating or somnambulistic eating, is essentially a form of sleepwalking. What is unique, however, is that patients will report unexplained weight gain or evidence of eating in their sleep (crumbs in the bed, food wrappers from food they cannot remember eating, and the like). The way to deal with sleep eating is similar to how we deal with sleepwalking. It begins with treating any underlying sleep conditions like sleep apnea, stopping the use of offending medications like the "Z" drugs, and, sometimes, the using different medications (such as certain antiseizure meds).

Sleep restriction therapy, along with stimulus control therapy, is a major part of cognitive behavioral therapy for insomnia (see "CBT-I—Cognitive behavioral therapy for insomnia"), which is a group of behavioral changes we recommend to improve chronic insomnia. While this may not sound like fun, it can be a very effective treatment when paired with other improvements and/or medication. Online programs have recently become available, but I recommend that it be done under the guidance of a CBT-I therapist.

The easiest way to explain how sleep restriction therapy works is through an extreme example. Let's say a person gets into bed at 8:00 p.m. but doesn't fall asleep until midnight. Then midnight comes, and he's waking up every hour and finally gets out of bed at 8:00 a.m. He's in bed from 8:00 p.m. to 8:00 a.m.—a total of twelve hours—but really is only sleeping six. Why is this a problem? Because when people spend too much time in bed, their brain starts to get conditioned; in effect, it is saying, "This bed is not my place of sleep. This is my place of worry. This is my place of frustration. This is my place of anxiety." The bottom line is it becomes a perpetuating factor in chronic insomnia, and we need to fix it (see "Precipitating, and perpetuating factors of chronic insomnia: the "3P" model").

We fix this is by retraining the brain, which sleep restriction helps us to do. In this example, I would instruct the patient not to get into bed until 1:00 a.m. and then to wake up at 7:00 a.m. (no matter what). This is not meant to be a punishment, but it means that the patient can only sleep a maximum of six hours at night. Over a period of a few weeks, his brain begins to restructure itself. It "knows" that it is only allowed six hours in bed, so it has to make the most of the time it is given. Patients will go through several days of being sleep deprived and tired during the day. To make things worse, I tell them they cannot nap.

The first couple of weeks can be hell, with patients likely cursing my name, but sleep restriction therapy usually works if they stick to it. While it can incredibly effective, there are risks. People with bipolar disorder, for example, may end up in a full-blown manic episode as a result of sleep restriction. Or someone could be drowsy when they drive due to sleep deprivation. Again, if you decide to embark on sleep restriction therapy, it is my opinion that you make sure that your doctor, a sleep specialist, or a therapist is aware of the course you are taking.

Sleep stages. The two main stages of sleep are rapid eye movement (REM) sleep and non-rapid eye movement (non-REM) sleep. These alternate during the night, giving us sleep cycles and resulting in our sleep architecture. (See "REM sleep" and "NREM, or non-REM sleep" for more information.)

Sleep starts are very common (and benign) involuntary twitches that occur just as a person is beginning to fall asleep, similar to a hiccup. They have several names, ranging from hypnic jerk and hypnagogic jerk, to sleep twitch and night start. They can cause the person to awaken suddenly for a brief time, which may interrupt sleep, and they also may also be accompanied by a falling sensation. Sleep starts are not dangerous in and of themselves, but they may be a sign of poor sleep quality or quantity.

Sleep talking (somniloquy). As many as two-thirds of people have, at one time or another, talked in their sleep. Like confusional arousals and other similar disorders, sleep talking is benign, but if it happens frequently and/or disrupts a person's sleep (or their bed partner's sleep), it might be useful to have an evaluation to rule out any serious conditions like sleep apnea. Also, there is *no* data suggesting that what a person says in their sleep has any relevance to deep-seated thoughts or desires that the person may be holding in their mind. In other words, despite what soap operas would have us believe, people who talk in their sleep are not necessarily revealing any deep, dark secrets.

Sleep terrors (night terrors) are comprised of episodes of loud screams and what seems like extreme panic. They typically occur in children. What surprises most people is that the child is not having a nightmare. In fact, he or she usually has no recollection of the event at all. The parents, however, are the ones to suffer, as the blood-curdling screams will almost always wake them from sleep.

Following a nightmare, a child will give a very detailed account of the dream and seek to be consoled. By contrast, in sleep terrors, the child is very difficult to wake up; he or she is in deep sleep, N3 sleep, and thus has sleep inertia.

As with sleepwalking, children tend to outgrow sleep terrors, but they can impact adults as well. If they happen frequently, one technique would be to wake the patient preemptively, typically fifteen to thirty minutes before the sleep terrors usually take place. When they are severe (especially when present in adults), an overnight sleep test would be useful to look for sleep apnea or other sleep disruptors. In some cases, medication or other treatment is needed.

Sleep trackers. Many people find it helpful to invest in a sleep tracker, which is one of the new types of high-tech items now on the market. These devices purport to monitor your sleep patterns, producing a clearer picture of exactly how much quality and quantity of sleep you're getting.

Examples include a Fitbit or an Apple Watch fitness tracker that you can wear at nighttime. Wearable tech of this sort can track a person's movements throughout the day and night by using an algorithm that shows whether the person is in deep sleep, light sleep, or is awake. It's not a perfect measurement, but it helps patients keep track of things and gets them more engaged in their health, so in that regard, I like them. On the other hand, these technologies are not able to definitively measure the quality of sleep and other key specifics, so we have to be careful when we are evaluating for an actual sleep disorder.

Sleepwalking (somnambulism) is common in childhood, but it's only seen in about 4 percent of adults. Non-REM stage 2 (N2) is the baseline of our sleep, N3 is very deep sleep, and sleepwalking occurs as we transition from N2 sleep into N3 sleep. The reason children experience sleepwalking more often than adults is because they tend to spend more time in N3. While sleepwalking is mostly benign, it can be a signal that something is wrong. It could be a warning that a condition is present that leads to partial awakenings (e.g., sleep apnea). Similarly, if someone spends a lot of time in N3—either from being chronically sleep deprived or from an irregular sleep schedule—there is a higher likelihood of sleepwalking. Some medications like nonbenzo Z drugs have been reported to cause sleepwalking.

As I discussed in *Let's Talk About Sleep*, one of my favorite movies is the comedy *Step Brothers*. In it, the lead characters are forty-somethings who, among other problems, suffer from sleepwalking. It is very funny to see in the movie and, believe or not, there is some truth to how it is portrayed.

During sleepwalking, certain areas of the brain are shut off while others are still working (see "Anatomy of sleep"). The frontal lobes are the areas of the brain that provide a "filter" so that behavior is socially acceptable. When people sleepwalk, the frontal lobes are still asleep but other areas of the brain are awake. The parietal lobes, which controls our automatic actions such as walking, opening a door, or even operating a car, are still active. This allows people to move about in their environment without actually knowing what they're doing, and you can see how this would be a problem. People say that one should never wake a sleepwalker, and the reason for this is that since the frontal lobes are asleep, any kind of sudden movement (like what would occur when abruptly awakening a person) may be perceived as a threat—also, the filter has been turned off. As a result, the sleepwalker could do harm to himself or someone else.

What can one do about sleepwalking? If there is a possibility of another sleep condition (again, like sleep apnea), it should be addressed first. But the key thing to focus on is bedtime safety, including locked doors and windows, taking the knobs off ovens and stoves, and so on. Sometimes medications may be the answer, whether that is to eliminate or change it. In the case of the Z drugs, changing to another sleep aide may help. For the bed partner, guiding the sleepwalker back to bed with reassuring statements is helpful as well.

Snoring. When someone has a tight airway—either from nasal congestion, a deviated septum, fat tissue around the neck, a genetically tight airway, a large tongue, or any combination of the above—the result can be snoring, which is simply a vibration of these tissues. Snoring of its own accord is not considered dangerous but can be associated with obstructive sleep apnea (see "OSA—Obstructive sleep apnea").

In most cases, any treatment that improves sleep apnea will also improve snoring, but there are options that just treat snoring. Breathe Right nasal strips, a mouth guard (SnoreRx is a good one), or even ENT surgery—nasal turbinate reduction or "UPPP" (see Uvulopala-topharyngoplasty [UPPP])—can be helpful. And just like with sleep apnea, avoiding alcohol and smoking (especially before bed), avoiding sleeping flat on your back, and getting rid of excess weight are useful.

Sodium oxybate. See "Gamma hydroxybutyrate"

Stimulant medications are classes of medications used to treat excessive daytime sleepiness. They include non-amphetamines such as Ritalin/Concerta (methylyphenidate) and Focalin (dexmethylpheni-date). Amphetamine-based stimulants include Adderall (amphetamine/dextroamphetamine) and Vyvanse (lisdexamfetamine). While they work for a variety of conditions such as narcolepsy and idiopathic hypersomnia, they can have effects on the blood pressure and heart rate, and they can be addictive.

Stimulus control therapy is the age-old rule of only using the bed for sleep and sex. But we incorporate into it what I call the "twenty-minute rule." Let's say someone gets into bed and cannot get to sleep. Without looking at a clock, if they feel twenty minutes or so has gone by and they are not any closer to sleep, I advise them to get up out of bed, go to another area of the house—for example, the living room—and do a relaxing activity.

A relaxing activity could be a mindfulness or guided meditation (my favorite), reading a book on paper, listening to an audio book or soft music, taking a warm bath, sitting quietly with some candles, and so on. The principle here is to relax without utilizing the blue light devices we have come to rely on (see "Blue light"). In fact, the TV, tablet, computer, smartphone, and all aspects of the work environment should be out of the bedroom or, at least, out of the bed space.

Once people are feeling more relaxed, they can get back into bed, try again, and do this as many times as it takes. The idea here is to retrain your brain into thinking that "my bed is my place of sleep, not my place of rumination, frustration, and so on." In this way, it is like the other form of CBT-I: sleep restriction therapy. And, as it goes with CBT-I, it can be frustrating in the beginning, but it's very effective over the long term.

Stress (particularly chronic stress), whether it be from home or the job, can lead to an unhealthy balance in which the body is in a state of inflammation and fight or flight hormones are being released chronically. These issues can be followed by the negative consequences of poor sleep, weight gain, and an overall sense of a lack of wellbeing. We have been designed to have the body use stress hormones like cortisol occasionally, but not when their use is a regular occurrence.

All this may be compounded by a lack of physical exercise. Humans are meant to move. When we don't, it is as if our bodies have not burned off the excess energy, and it can make it more difficult to fall asleep at night. Multiple studies have shown that simply adding twenty to thirty minutes of regular exercise a day can have a profound effect on insomnia. I usually tell my patients to get cardio exercise in the morning and then to meditate at night. This is a powerful combination that burns off excess body energy and quiets the mind.

To sum up, chronic stress can lead to poor sleep, which then makes it more difficult for the body to process the stress; this can lead to changes in exercise and diet that then make everything worse, keeping the vicious cycle going. Especially during the recent COVID-19 pandemic, where people have been and continue to spend excessive amounts of time indoors, chronic stress has become even more prevalent and even more important to address.

Sunlight. It should come as no surprise that sunlight is our strongest zeitgeber, a German word which literally means "time giver." We must rely on sunlight to keep our circadian rhythm and internal body clock in check. Sunlight is so important because it shuts down the production of melatonin, thus cutting off the signal that tells us to sleep.

At various points throughout this book, I recommend getting sunlight (around twenty minutes) in the morning (along with exercise) and then, at night, allowing melatonin to do its thing by shutting off smartphones, TVs, and all other screens thirty to sixty minutes before bed. Of course, when I say "get sunlight," I do not mean to stare at the sun but to simply be outside, or by a window, allowing the sunlight to shine on you. This is using light to your advantage. It is a big part of improving sleep hygiene.

Surgical options for obstructive sleep apnea. There are several entries throughout this book detailing some surgical options for OSA: the MMA, the Inspire device, and the UPPP. However, for the sake of completeness, I want to mention two more here: hyoid bone suspension and rapid maxillary expansion.

The hyoid bone is a U-shaped bone in the neck located above the Adam's apple. It has attachments to muscles of the tongue as well as other muscles and soft tissues that surround the airway, but it is quite mobile and not firmly anchored in position. A hyoid suspension repositions the hyoid bone toward the jaw, which improves the stability of the airway and may improve OSA.

Rapid maxillary expansion is a procedure mostly used in children with OSA (this book is for adults, but I wanted to mention it here anyway). An orthodontist will place temporary hardware over several of the rear teeth—once in place, the brace is further adjusted over time by a parent with a special key. These adjustments will gradually widen the hard palate, which is the roof of the mouth, as well as the floor of the nasal passage. Thus, when widened, the space through which air moves is increased, and this may reduce the collapse of the airway that causes OSA.

Taping the mouth closed with surgical tape is a do-it-yourself treatment that some people say helps them get a good night's sleep. Here's why: if you are not able to use your mouth to breathe, your nose will suffice. Some data suggest that nasal breathing increases nitric oxide production in the sinuses, which may reduce inflammation and lead to improved sleep, improved memory, and an overall increase in immune system function. Some people have reported that—just from this change—they wake up feeling more rested, without a dry mouth or a sore throat.

At the same time, other data suggest that mouth breathing is not only *not* good for us but that it can contribute to sleep apnea, high blood pressure, and asthma. And some experts suggest that mouth breathing can lead to tooth decay, owing to a change in oral bacteria and from dryness.

While I would not necessarily suggest mouth taping as a treatment for most sleep problems, it is worth a try for those who prefer natural or non-harmful remedies to help improve their sleep. It should not, however, be used alone as a treatment for sleep apnea. For more details, go to www.everydayhealth.com/sleep/mouth-taping-cheapest-life-hack -better-sleep.

Technology (new approaches to improving sleep) has long had a dramatic impact on the treatment of sleep disorders. Continuous positive airway pressure (CPAP), invented more than thirty-five years ago, revolutionized the treatment of snoring and sleep apnea, a condition that previously required drastic surgical measures to resolve.

The future of sleep in the age of technology is on everyone's mind these days, and the business behind it is booming. The number of products designed to enhance sleep grows on a day-by-day basis. Today's lineup includes hundreds of smartphone apps, wearable technology like fitness trackers, smart beds, mattresses, and a variety of external devices that monitor what goes on in the bedroom. The list also includes devices designed to optimize the sleep environment by regulating light, noise, temperature, and humidity. Additionally, it includes interventions that treat snoring, sleep apnea, circadian disorders, and insomnia. While there is no one answer for everyone, the internet is obviously the place to go for a look at what's available and where the future of sleep in the age of technology is heading.

Teeth grinding and/or jaw clenching are known as bruxism, a condition that can have various causes; the most common are stress, anxiety, and untreated sleep apnea. If a patient is sent to me by a dentist, I will usually start by doing a sleep test. If the problem turns out to be sleep apnea, I will attempt to treat it with CPAP or an oral device (MAD). If the test is negative, I may suggest a psychiatric evaluation or therapy, meditation, or other de-stressing techniques. This approach doesn't cover all of grinding, but it's a good start. Regardless of the cause, a dentist may make a mouth guard to protect the teeth, which can be used with a CPAP if needed or combined with an MAD.

TIB—time in bed—is just what it sounds like: how much time we spend in bed, whether asleep or not. It is part of the sleep efficiency calculation.

Tips for healthy sleep (from National Institutes of Health):

- Stick to a schedule. Go to bed and wake up at the same time each day. To make sure this program works, set an alarm not only for your morning wake up but also for bedtime each of the seven days a week.
- Cardio exercise at least twenty to thirty minutes every day, ideally in the morning, but not within three hours of bedtime.

- Avoid caffeine and nicotine totally—if that's not possible, then within eight hours of bedtime.
- Avoid alcohol before bed.
- Avoid large meals and beverages late at night.
- Avoid medicines that delay or disrupt your sleep.
- Do not nap after 3:00 p.m.
- Relax before bedtime. Make reading, listening to music, or other relaxing activities a part of your bedtime ritual.
- Take a hot bath before bed.
- Make sure your bedroom is dark, cool, and free of cell phones, TVs, or other devices that might be a distraction.
- Try to get outside into the sunlight for at least thirty minutes a day.
- If you are still awake twenty minutes after you get into bed, get up and do a relaxing activity until you feel sleepy.

Tongue stimulation for apnea. A new methodology to treat snoring and mild obstructive sleep apnea (OSA) has recently emerged and been cleared by the FDA. It is a prescription tongue muscle stimulation device, called eXciteOSA, approved for people eighteen years and over. This device is purported to work by improving tongue muscle function while awake and, over time, may prevent the tongue from falling backward and obstructing the airway during sleep.

The eXciteOSA device, made by Signifier Medical Technologies, is essentially a silicone mouthpiece with four electrodes that are placed above and below the tongue. It works by delivering muscle stimulations electronically with rest periods in between, and it's recommended to be used for twenty minutes once per day for six weeks, and then once per week after that.

It is important to note that this is not approved for those with high levels of OSA, those with pacemakers or other forms of implanted pacing electrodes, those who are pregnant (it's simply not been studied in them), those with ulcerations in or around the mouth, and those who have dental and orthodontic hardware like braces. In fact, a dental exam is recommended before starting, as the most common side effects from eXciteOSA include excessive salivation, tongue or tooth discomfort, and a sensation of jaw tightness.

Tonsils are organs in the back of our throats that serve as the immune system's first line of defense against ingested or inhaled substances. They do this through the use of special capture cells called microfold cells (M cells) on their surface. When the tonsils are inflamed and enlarged, the condition is called tonsillitis. If the condition becomes chronic, the tonsils can become so enlarged that they affect breathing at night (see "OSA—Obstructive sleep apnea"). Removing the tonsils is common in children, but it's much less so in adults, with the reason being the risk of serious bleeding. As part of the UPPP surgery (see "Uvulopalatopharyn-goplasty [UPPP]") for sleep apnea, the tonsils may be removed, along with the uvula and part of the soft palate. This, in theory, would reduce snoring and the apnea itself, although this does not work very well in practice. An ENT doctor would be the first stop to make if tonsils are a major problem for you.

Trauma-associated sleep disorder (TSD). Nightmares and disruptive nocturnal behaviors are part of REM behavior disorder (see "REM behavior disorder [RBD]"). However, a newly described condition called TSD is a little different. Here, there is a traumatic experience or extreme stress combined with periods of sleep disruption and/or deprivation. Unlike RBD, TSD is thought to be caused by hyperarousal, which is an increased fight or flight response to a minimal threat—a loud sound, for example. This hyperarousal distinguishes TSD from RBD, in which we are more concerned about an impending neurologic illness. TSD is still a "young" condition, and in time (as more research is done), we will understand more about it.

TST—total sleep time—is a measure of how much we actually sleep, not how long we spend in bed. Like time in bed (TIB), it is part of the sleep efficiency calculation.

$\mathcal{U}$

Upper airway anatomy. Patients often ask where their obstructive sleep apnea (OSA) came from, and the answer in many cases is a combination of factors. Weight, being a man, getting older, or being postmenopausal in a woman are all risk factors; however, sometimes none of these fully explains the presence of OSA. The upper airway—which consists of the tongue, the soft tissue, the uvula, the tonsils, and the place where the palate sits in the back of the throat—are among the main factors.

Sometimes, problems with upper airway anatomy is demonstrated during a procedure like a colonoscopy. After the anesthesia starts to work, the doctor may notice loud snoring or even stoppages of breathing, which are a result of a tight airway being made tighter when the muscles are relaxed. Many patients come to me as a result of this type of scenario. The bottom line is that being thin does *not* mean that a person cannot have OSA. It is the upper airway anatomy that dictates this.

Upper airway resistance syndrome (UARS) is a much less well-known condition than snoring and obstructive sleep apnea (OSA), but it is just as important.

When the airway is wide open, there are no problems with breathing during sleep. When the airway is a little bit tight, you have snoring. When it is more than a little tight, you have upper airway resistance. And when the airway is closed off, you have OSA. Thus, UARS falls in the middle between snoring and OSA, where the airway is not closed off enough for us to consider this a case of OSA, but it's also not considered normal. An overnight sleep test (PSG) would be the ideal way to diagnose UARS, especially if a home sleep test was negative; it is more precise and can show how the brain responds to the tightened airway (i.e., the increased upper airway resistance) by having what I call mini awakenings (arousals) through the night.

How do OSA and UARS differ? They sound like they are similar conditions and should have similar symptoms, but this is not the case. OSA patients are tired, have chopped-up sleep, and high blood pressure (See "OSA—Obstructive sleep apnea"). People with UARS have a different set of symptoms: they are anxious, may have low blood pressure, and may have fatigue as opposed to sleepiness.

Despite the differences, the treatment is very similar. You've got to keep the airway open, whether with a CPAP, an oral device, or whatever. Unfortunately, since UARS is not as well-understood or as prominent as OSA, some patients may have trouble getting a doctor to prescribe treatment and an insurance company to approve the treatment. Interested readers are urged to learn about UARS and discuss it with your doctor if any of this hits home.

Uvula. The uvula is the little "punching bag" that hangs in the back of the throat (as it is often portrayed in cartoons); it plays a role in collecting dust, microbes, and other debris, so they don't end up in our lungs. It also helps create certain sounds, but it is by no means a necessary organ. In fact, its most notable "function" is that it is the part of the upper airway that vibrates during snoring. Thus, removing the uvula with a procedure known as a UPPP (see "Uvulopalatopharyngoplasty [UPPP]") reduces snoring.

Uvulopalatopharyngoplasty (UPPP) is a procedure whereby an ENT surgeon will remove excess tissue in the throat—namely, the uvula (see "Uvula") and the soft palate (and sometimes any tonsil tissue that is present). Since the organ that causes snoring (i.e., the uvula) is removed, this can be used as a definitive treatment for snoring. But the data and clinical experience suggest that a UPPP might not be useful enough for a significant case of obstructive sleep apnea (OSA); in those cases, use of CPAP or a dental device (MAD) would likely still be needed.

Virtual appointments with a sleep doctor. During the writing of this book, the COVID-19 pandemic (see "COVID-19 and sleep") was affecting the world at large. One positive result was that virtual appointments for outpatient doctors became more prominent, as people were unwilling to travel to in-person appointments on buses or trains or to sit in busy waiting rooms.

A virtual appointment is sometimes called a virtual visit or video visit, and it can be done through a number of services (Doximity and Zoom being among the most popular). Some areas of medicine preclude this service as a viable option, as a physical exam needs to take place; however, it is fortunate that in sleep medicine we can usually get by without one. During a virtual visit, we can find out a great deal about a patient's symptoms and review test results and treatment options.

One question we are frequently asked is whether someone who uses continuous positive airway pressure (CPAP) might be able to have a meaningful virtual appointment, and the answer is a strong yes. CPAP machines nowadays transmit data through wireless services, which allows doctors to see their patient's data in a second by signing on to the CPAP manufacturer's portal. If your doctor or health care system allows for virtual appointments, you should see it as a good thing.

W

Wakefulness means consciousness, and an entire book could be devoted to this seemingly simple statement. However, for our purposes, being awake and alert reflects the interplay of multiple neurotransmitters in the brain, including orexin (hypocretin). When orexin is deficient, narcolepsy results (see "Narcolepsy").

Wake promoting agents are classes of medications that are considered to be less harsh in terms of blood pressure and heart rate elevation as compared to traditional stimulants. They include Provigil (modafinil), Nuvigil (armodafinil), Sunosi (solriamfetol), and Wakix (pitalosant).

Wake time consistency. Being consistent with the time we are awake is one of the most important things we can do for our sleep health. Our brains need to know that a particular window of time (say, 11:00 p.m. to 7:00 a.m.) is our time for sleep. When we deviate from this schedule— like sleeping late on the weekends—we can throw our internal clock off, and this can lead to trouble falling asleep at night.

Weighted blankets are heavy blankets that often aid in sleep and reduce anxiety. Their history began as therapeutic tools to aid people with neuropsychological conditions, such as autism spectrum disorders and dementia. In the late 1990s, weighted blankets were used by occupational therapists as a coping device for patients with special needs; they became part of what is known as sensory integration therapy and were used to help people with autism. Weighted blankets are now widespread and common in their use as a home remedy for insomnia.

White noise machines generate steady, continuous sounds intended to block out clanky radiators, barking dogs, sirens, a neighbor's TV, late-night parties, and other similar sounds that might keep us awake at night. The machines come in many different sizes, shapes, and prices. Designed to calm the listener, the noise they generate often resembles a rushing waterfall, wind blowing through the trees, and other natural sounds. Studies have shown that white noise machines can lead to better sleep.

Why We Sleep

> What probing deep
> Has ever solved the mystery of sleep?
>
> —Thomas Aldrich (1836–1907), "Human Ignorance"

Scientists have been trying for centuries to determine why the brain needs to disconnect from the environment for hours every day. And while the *why* in the question is still a scientific mystery, there are several facts about sleep that make us know it is vital for survival. The need for sleep is present in essentially all animals, and it has persisted in evolution even though it does not seemingly help in any way (during sleep, animals cannot search for food, eat, procreate, etc.). We know that sleep is needed for survival, but it still does not explain the *why*. As I have said, no one knows the answer, but some of our most brilliant minds have put forth theories. Here are a few of the more interesting ones:

- Conservation of energy.
- Cellular recovery/repair.
- Oxidative stress. As organisms move through their daily lives, the metabolism of cells leads to the formation of what are called "free radicals" (oxidative stress) that can, over time, lead to damage. It is thought that sleep combats this with its antioxidant properties.
- Neural network reorganization. Sleep strengthens certain connections in the brain while "pruning down" those that are not considered as important.
- The glymphatic system (see "Glymphatic system").

- Mental health. Symptoms of insomnia commonly coexist with depression and anxiety. Moreover, it has been demonstrated that acute sleep deprivation increases risk-taking behavior and impairs the ability to integrate emotion and cognition to guide moral judgments.

A great deal has also been published on the effects of sleep and sleep loss on cardiovascular health, inflammation, metabolic/endocrine function, carcinogenesis, and athletic performance. Currently, one of the biggest issues under discussion is how sleep affects the immune system. We know that chronically poor sleep can increase the risk of infection, and this has particular importance given the COVID-19 pandemic.

Yawning

> If you cough, sneeze, sigh, or yawn, do it not loud but privately; and speak not in your yawning, but put your handkerchief or hand before your face and turn aside.
>
> —George Washington

Just like with sleeping, everyone yawns. Yawning is a reflex action in which the lungs take air in and the eardrums stretch. Man is certainly not the only creature to yawn; turtles, birds, dogs, cats, and less advanced species have been known to do it. Even fetuses have been shown to yawn (as has been seen on an ultrasound). According to Aristotle, "Like a donkey urinates when he sees or hears another donkey do it, so also man yawn seeing someone else do it." This is a truism for sure, as we have all experienced this at one time or another. But what is the cause? Believe it or not, no one really knows why we yawn, though there are some proposed ideas.

Some texts have described yawning as an effort to open up the tiny air sacs in our lungs, called alveoli, and prevent their collapse and subsequent breathing trouble. Another concept states that yawning helps to cool the brain. Yawning has been shown to increase blood return to the heart, and it has been thought to play a role in taking in oxygen and getting rid of carbon dioxide.

Sometimes, yawning can be altered as a result of medical issues (such as diabetes, stroke, or adrenal conditions) or in those with immunosuppression. Nervousness or a nervous tic can also lead to yawning.

Research suggests that contagious yawning may be a sign of empathy, but that is up for debate. The brain has what are called mirror neurons, which are responsible for imitation behaviors from one person to another; this is thought to be at the heart of contagious yawning as well. One of my favorite shows, *MythBusters* on the Discovery Channel, tried to test this idea. They found that yawning was indeed contagious, but these results have been questioned. In certain neurological and psychiatric disorders, such as schizophrenia and autism, people have a reduced ability to read others. Because of this, the contagious yawn may not be seen.

Yawning is a very complex topic. While the data may put some people to sleep, the fact that we don't know why we yawn keeps researchers up at night.

Yoga. The word *yoga* comes from Sanskrit. It originated in India in roughly 3000 BC and literally means "union." Essentially, yoga is a combination of practices, poses/postures, and rituals that use mental, physical, and spiritual rituals to improve fitness, increase relaxation, and relieve stress. The fact that yoga is not only a simple physical exercise but also has a meditative and spiritual basis makes it a wonderful addition for any patient who is looking to naturally improve his or her sleep. Like many of the ideas discussed in this book, the practice of yoga is something I recommend to help with insomnia (and sleep in general), even though the data are not rigorous. But, as I always say, if it doesn't hurt and *may* help, it's worth a try.

$\mathcal{Z}$

Zzz. It is serendipitous that we end our journey with *Z*, the letter most associated with sleep. *Zzz* is an onomatopoeia, which is a word that imitates or resembles the sound that it describes; a great example would be animal noises, such as *oink*. It is thought *Zzz* was written as a representation of snoring in this fashion, but the history is unclear. Famed American author Henry David Thoreau was the first writer to represent certain sounds with the letter *Z*, but in his case, he was writing about the sound of crickets, not snoring.

Anyway, the purpose of this book is to help you, the reader, become familiar with all aspects of sleep and sleep health. But if there is one takeaway, it is this: sleep is vital for both our day-to-day functioning as well as our long-term health. It is important to get both *quality* sleep and *quantity* of sleep, and if there is any possibility of a sleep disorder in yourself or a loved one, I urge you to speak to a medical professional.

That said, we can't force ourselves to sleep. I always say that sleep is like love: you can't make either one happen, but what you *can* do is improve yourself and your situation and let nature take over. It is my hope that this book, in some small way, will help you do just that.

I leave you with this thought. It was written by Paulo Coehlo, author of *The Alchemist*—one of my favorite books. And while it does not really have anything to do with sleep health per se, it does recount one significant theme that I have tried to highlight throughout this book, namely, when it comes to any important desire—whether it be to sleep better, to improve your health, to live in that dream house, or to get that dream job—sticking to it is all that matters.

Before a dream is realized, the Soul of the World tests everything that was learned along the way. It does this not because it is evil, but so that we can, in addition to realizing our dreams, master the lessons we've learned as we've moved toward that dream. That's the point at which most people give up. It's the point at which, as we say in the language of the desert, one dies of thirst just when the palm trees have appeared on the horizon.

ABOUT THE AUTHORS

Daniel A. Barone, MD, is currently the associate medical director of the Weill Cornell Center for Sleep Medicine, an associate professor of Clinical Neurology at Weill Cornell Medical College, and a neurologist at New York-Presbyterian/Weill Cornell Medical Center. He specializes in the evaluation and management of patients with all forms of sleep disorders, including sleep apnea, restless legs syndrome, insomnia, and narcolepsy. He is certified by the American Board of Psychiatry and Neurology in both neurology and sleep medicine. He is a member of the American Academy of Neurology and is a fellow of both the American Academy of Sleep Medicine and the American Neurological Association.

Dr. Barone is the first author of multiple peer-reviewed publications on a variety of topics in sleep medicine and has appeared in several media pieces. His first book, *Let's Talk About Sleep*, was published in 2018.

Lawrence A. Armour is a freelance writer/editor who focused on business, finance, and medicine during his twenty years at Time Inc., *Fortune*, and *The Wall Street Journal*. He also spent ten years in communications at IBM and American Express, and he is the author of nine books. The first, *The Young Millionaires,* was followed by *Profits on Wall Street, Investing for Profit, How to Survive a Bear Market,* and *Managing to Succeed.* Other books include *How to Make Your Money Make Money,* written with Arthur Levitt Jr.; *The RealAge Workout,* written with Dr. Michael F. Roizen; *Manhattan Eye, Ear and Throat Hospital—150 Years of Visionary History,* written with Dr. Paul N. Orloff and Dr. Richard P. Gibralter; and *Let's Talk About Sleep,* written with Dr. Daniel A. Barone.

Armour is a graduate of Dartmouth and holds an MBA from Northwestern University.